Be a Loser!

Be a Loser!

Lose Inches Fast—No Diet

GREER CHILDERS
with Bobbie Katz

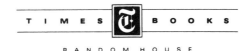

TIMES 🅣 BOOKS

RANDOM HOUSE

New York

No book, including this one, can ever replace the advice of a qualified physician.
Please consult your doctor before beginning this or any other exercise program.

Originally published in hardcover by Times Books,
a division of Random House, Inc., in 1998.

Library of Congress Cataloging-in-Publication Data
Childers, Greer.
Be a loser! : lose inches fast—no diet /
by Greer Childers with Bobbie Katz.
p.   cm.
ISBN 0-8129-3141-6
1. Exercise.   2. Physical fitness.   3. Weight loss.   I. Katz,
Bobbie.   II. Title.
GV481.C614 1998
613.7′1—dc21   97-45945

Random House website address: www.randomhouse.com
Printed in the United States of America

24689753

First Paperback Edition

Interior design by Robert Bull Design

To my three sons—Jeff, Ray, and Paul—whose coming into the world made me one of the happiest . . . and heaviest . . . people I have ever known. Thanks for being your wonderful selves and for contributing to the inch-by-inch process that made this book possible. And thanks also to Linda, my terrific daughter-in-law, who is happy that I brought Jeff into the world, too! You're all the true heavyweights in my life!

CONTENTS

What do all these people have in common? Ivana Trump. Wayne Newton. Engelbert Humperdinck. Phyllis McGuire of the fabulous McGuire Sisters. Steve Rossi of the famous comedy team Allen & Rossi. Danny Gans, comic impressionist.

Dr. Daniel Mowrey, famed scientist, Ph.D., and author. Barry Markman, M.D., noted board-certified plastic surgeon and researcher of adipose tissue. Dr. Art Davis, family practice physician and former chief of staff and chairman of the Department of Family Practices for JFK Hospital in California. Dr. Gary Halversen, radiologist. Dr. Carolyn DeMarco, author and women's health journalist. Tony Martinez, U.S. national karate expert and Golden Glove boxer. Markus Daxl, certified personal trainer and former Mr. Heavyweight Nevada.

Burton Goldberg, author of the best-selling *Alternative Medicine: The Definitive Guide*. Doug Terry, former vice president, Morris Air/president Funjet International. Mark Faler, vice president, Dain Rauscher (the nation's tenth largest securities firm). Libby Gardon, president, Consumer Health Organization of Canada. Doug and Krystyna Widdifield, president/CEO Yu-ccan International, manufacturer and distributor of natural health and environmental products. Gary Smith, owner/CEO Health Rider. Amanda Borghese, cosmetics icon.

Models. Former Miss and Mrs. Americas. A former Miss Universe.

And millions of everyday people. Can't figure out what they all have in common? Well, they're all LOSERS! Collectively they've all lost untold inches and weight on the hottest fitness program sweeping the country: BodyFlex.

I'm probably one of the biggest losers of all time. I went from a size 14–16 to a size 4–6 in ninety days using this unique method. I'm Greer Childers, the creator of BodyFlex, which is based on a principle of burning excess body fat and building lean muscle mass by utilizing a specialized accelerated aerobic breathing technique combined with isometric, isotonic, and stretch positions that oxygenate the cells. The result? Aerobic conditioning, greater vitality, and inch loss fast. In fact, I've had thousands of clients lose 4 to 14 inches the first week from the waist, thighs, hips, and stomach. All in just fifteen minutes a day—and with no dieting.

Okay, by now I can practically hear you screaming, "Four to fourteen inches in one week in just fifteen minutes a day just from breathing!? Now, how stupid is that! You've gotta be kidding." I completely understand your skepticism—I was there myself. But give me a few minutes; by the time you've finished reading this book and tried Body-Flex, you, too, will be a believer—and a loser!

We've all been beaten over the head with the idea that we must exercise, we must eat right, and we must not abuse our bodies if we want to maintain good health and have a longer, more vibrant life. The evidence is overwhelming that oxygen plays *the* key role in our health, well-being, and fitness level. In fact, in 1931, Dr. Otto Warburg won the Nobel Prize in medicine for discovering the cause of cancer. His award-winning work revealed that there is one prime cause of cancer: lack of oxygen to the cell. That alone should make us stand up and take notice.

I have spent the last dozen years doing research on the topic of oxygenation. From that research, I developed BodyFlex. I have taught this program to many physicians, respiratory therapists, cardiologists, and sports medicine physicians and my videotapes have been distributed in hospitals and clinics across the United States and Canada. I have just finished making an infomercial that will take this program to Europe and Asia. In August 1997, participants in a study lost an average of 8.4 inches total from their waist, hips, thighs, and arms in just two weeks. Body-Flex has been written about by noted scientist, author, and lecturer Dr. Daniel Mowrey in his book, *Fat Management: The Thermogenic Factor,* and by medical expert Dr. Carolyn DeMarco in her columns in various newspapers and publications throughout Canada. Many noted practitioners in the U.S. and Canada practice BodyFlex and give the Body-Flex tapes to their patients. BodyFlex has also been used in Salt Lake City, Utah, as therapy for asthma, allergy, and cystic fibrosis.

But the greatest testimonial to the power of Body-Flex has come from the general public. To date, I have sold more than 3 million sets of videotapes throughout the United States and Canada on the Home Shopping Network and QVC. BodyFlex became the number one highest volume product on the Home Shopping Network in Canada. In this country, my second time on the Home Shopping Network, I was given the largest single order the network had ever given anyone in its history—70,000 sets of tapes— and I sold them out in four days. And, on QVC, which clocks success by dollars per minute, the average being $2,500 per minute, the last show I did for them I sold

$46,000 a minute—21,000 sets of tapes in 18 minutes. This kind of success tells me two things: first, there's a huge need for a doable exercise program that brings results fast; and second, when people find something that does the job, they spread the word. Every time I go on the air to talk about BodyFlex, I take phone calls from folks who have done the program and are thrilled by the results.

And that's the bottom line for me. I have a real commitment to others to make a difference in their lives just as this technique made a difference in mine. I get thousands of letters and phone calls from people BodyFlex has helped; some of those letters can be found in Chapter 9 of this book. While we all want to look good and be fit and firm, it's a sad fact that the reason most of us don't exercise is because we keep doing the same thing over and over and we don't see results. So we get discouraged and give up. We live in a society that thrives on instant gratification. If we can see with our own two eyes that something is working and working fast, that's motivation enough for us to keep going. That's why my program has been so successful. Very simply, it works.

Real Exercise for Real People

The key to BodyFlex is that it is designed for people of all ages and is something almost everyone can do, even if they have physical limitations. I, myself, am fifty-three years old. I don't want to have to bop down to some gym to compete with the twentysomething fitness gym bunnies. I've got clients in wheelchairs, clients with chronic illnesses. And a lot of folks who just basically wrote exercise out of their lives until they found BodyFlex. The fact is that 90 percent of the public doesn't exercise at all, so why do alleged exercise gurus insist on putting them through the roller, rocker, rider, cruncher syndrome? Most of us are lucky if we have enough energy to walk from the sofa to the kitchen—we live in a tired society. And most of us want to hear from someone who understands what it's like to go through a few pregnancies or see parts of your body head south as you get older. We want real exercise because we're real people. So shouldn't someone design a program for the masses? The answer is yes, and I've done it. That's exactly what BodyFlex is.

Facing Down the Skeptics

I've been winning over the eye-rollers for a long time. Initially, lots of people bucked me on it, both customers and colleagues. The biggest complaint was that I wasn't a Ph.D. or an exercise physiologist, so what did I know about exercise? At that time, I may not have known everything there was to know on the subject, but I certainly knew what I didn't want. I didn't want to be fat and I didn't want to be flabby. The one thing I knew for sure from the research I had done was that oxygen is what burns fat. So why would I want to submit my body to running and jumping and bouncing around just to increase the oxygen flow to burn fat when there was a way to do that without running myself ragged? BodyFlex only takes fifteen minutes a day to achieve maximum benefits for inch loss and fitness.

So the resistance I was encountering didn't matter because I knew what I was talking about—I had done my homework. I would tell anyone who taunted me, "Fine. Go home and don't do it. Because as smart as you are, whatever you've done all these years hasn't worked, and I'm standing up here at a size 4–6 telling you that I've found something that will work. If you think I'm a liar, go home." Of course, that motivated them into doing the program, and the results spoke for themselves.

I once had a particularly skeptical guy, a professional cyclist, come to one of my classes. His secretary had taken my class and he saw her getting more and more toned every day. When he asked her what she was doing, she replied, "BodyFlex. I'm breathing." Convinced this was a "scam," he showed up just to bust it wide open. "Well, I know this isn't going to work," he said very antagonistically to me. "I know my secretary's getting smaller, but she's probably dieting. And I know what endurance is at my level of exercise." He sat through the lecture and lesson, then left the class without even saying good-bye. A week later, he came back for part two—I have also developed an advanced BodyFlex technique—and his attitude was entirely changed.

"I've been a cyclist for twelve years," he told me, "and I know what my endurance is, how long I can ride, when I get tired, etcetera. I took seven minutes off my ride this last week—that's almost unheard of. For someone who has been riding for twelve years to be able to skim seven minutes off his ride is unbelievable. I came here for the wrong reasons and got the right results. I am impressed." After that, he became one of my biggest advocates and sent a lot of clients to me.

Likewise, when I first approached the Home Shopping Network in Canada two years ago, I was told by the fitness buyer, "We don't want any. Fitness tapes don't work;

the public doesn't like them." I said to him, "You don't know anything about this program. This is different." He replied, "Fitness is fitness." And I said to him, "You're going to have to tell me that to my face." So I hung up and drove over to the station, and managed to get myself into his office, where he told me to my face what he had told me on the phone. But I was relentless, and the poor guy finally said he would give me one chance to go on the air with a small order. He gave me five days, an hour at a time, to sell 1,700 sets of tapes. I sold them all in one day and with nothing more to sell, I had to go home. The proof is in the pudding. From that beginning, I've been winning over skeptics one at a time. And I know I can win you over.

You Too Can Be a Loser

I am a firm believer that if people understand, in simple terms, why and how something works, and how to do it properly, it makes all the difference in enabling them to achieve the maximum benefits. There are too many exercise programs out there where even the people behind them don't understand how they, or exercise in general for that matter, work. That is not the case with BodyFlex. That's why I've written this book. I want to educate you, in simple, easy-to-understand language, about the benefits of oxygen, which I call the non-medical miracle, in weight and inch loss and health. I want to show you how everything I say is backed up by medical research so you can feel secure in doing the workout—and maybe face down some of the eye-rollers you meet. I want to give you step-by-step instructions on the technique and workout so you'll feel as if you had a private training session with me. I want to show you how to extend the benefits of BodyFlex with good nutrition. Finally, I want to share with you some of the comments from and pictures of people like you and me, people who look good, feel good, and have improved their overall fitness level and health through BodyFlex.

I want you to be a loser, too. Let's get started.

Be a Loser!

1

■

Average American Women Don't Take Limos

I was an overweight, out-of-shape, tired, frustrated, depressed, almost-forty-year-old housewife married to a surgeon who was never home, and I had just recently given birth to my third ten-pound child.

And that was just the beginning of my problems.

I also hated myself. I hated my life, I hated the way I looked, and, most of all, I *really* hated all those young skinny nurses who worked in my husband's office. Oh yeah, I hated my husband, too.

Then, one day, while staring at my image in the mirror, taking in the side view and trying to convince myself that I really wasn't that heavy, that my eyeglasses just happened to have a wide-angle lens, I finally couldn't deny the truth that was staring me, at least peripherally, in the face. It suddenly hit me: My whole problem was that I had been looking at myself the wrong way. For the last several years, I simply had had my head on backwards.

Literally.

"Greer," I said aloud to myself, "your stomach is big and round and protruding and your butt is flat. If your head could just be turned around the other way, you'd have a perfect profile!"

If I could've pulled that off, it actually would also have solved a second problem. With all those cute young nurses around my husband, who developed a severe drooling condition every time he looked at a size 6, it occurred to me that having eyes in the back of my head wouldn't have been such a bad idea. But despite my unrealistic assessment of the situation, that day started me on a journey to try to find a solution and to get myself back into shape. Little did I know it was to be a long, expensive, and roundabout trip.

Don't Rats Run on Treadmills, Too?

I jogged a good part of the way—enough to go around the world three or four times, I estimated. That didn't work. I tried a little side-stepping, going to a few Jazzercise classes—the class was going left and I was going right and they were going forward and I was going back. That didn't work for me either.

But I didn't give up. I lifted weights, I did squats, and I bought a Butt Blaster and a Thighmaster and any other weight-loss apparatus anyone could possibly think of. I even hired a personal trainer. He designed a program just for me, which I did as I continued to lift weights, squat, butt-crunch, and squeeze my thighs around this odd-looking contraption. I was going to the trainer three to four times a week, paying $50 at a clip, and you guessed it— none of this produced any results. I wanted to get lean, I wanted my stomach to be flat, I wanted the lumps and bumps on my thighs to melt away, and I wanted my rear end to be firm. But at the end of three months, when I looked at myself in the mirror, I was bigger rather than smaller. Yes, my legs were firmer and more muscular, but they were bigger. Unfortunately, what I had spent a small fortune to do, as I learned later, was to build muscle under existing fat as opposed to burning the fat and toning the muscle simultaneously.

After this episode, I was so upset and distraught that I went on prescription diet pills. I'd get up in the morning and hit the ground running and I didn't even know where I was going, I was so nervous. I remember attending different gatherings and watching some of the women walk in and thinking, Gee, they look great. Look at their legs, look at their shapely physiques . . . and here I am, wearing a muu-muu designed by Omar the Tentmaker (better known as a "tent dress" to those of my generation) so that people won't know what is or isn't under here. The pills, of course, didn't work either.

It was during this time that I came to the conclusion that the person who developed the A-line skirt should have won the Nobel Prize for "Best Camouflage Technique Resulting in Saving Millions of Women in the World from Humiliation during the Battle of the Bulge." After the skirt hits the waist, it flares out and no one can see those parts of the body that go bump in the night. In fact, all I had in my wardrobe were A-line skirts, because I couldn't wear anything that was straight or the slightest bit tight.

So, there I was. I had done everything from jogging, running, walking, hopping, skipping, and jumping rope to turning myself into a pretzel, to no avail. I was relatively young, but I hated the way I looked more than ever, and the way I felt was even worse. I was so tired all the time that my husband, thinking there was something desperately wrong with me, had me tested for everything from tuberculosis to leukemia. I had no get-up-and-go, barely possessing enough energy to get up from the couch to go into the kitchen and get a drink of water (I drank it warm to conserve the energy involved in pulling back the handle on the ice tray to release the cubes) and then go back to the couch and flop down again. In terms of being a couch potato, I was definitely mashed.

When you've tried every conventional method of weight loss and nothing works, when you hate the way you look and feel, when you've gotten to the point where it all seems so hopeless, it stands to reason that you might feel, as I did, that it's time to move on to the next step—antidepressants. Thanks to the pills, I couldn't eat . . . but I went around in circles, exercising and jogging and jogging and exercising. Nothing made any difference in my weight, my energy level, my mental attitude, or my appearance. I was still inclined to sue the city of Salt Lake for building the sidewalk too close to my butt. I decided I was going in the wrong direction altogether. And I was now becoming even more desperate.

But which way to turn? All I knew is what I wanted. I wanted what everyone else wanted. I wanted to look good, I wanted to feel good. I was tired of being tired—I got up tired, I went to work tired, I came home tired, I went to bed tired. I was dragging around all the time, pulling lots of flab around with me. And despite all my best efforts, a size 14 was now too tight. That signaled the end for me.

Jealousy: Always a Good Motivator

One day I met up with my next-door neighbor, with whom I used to chew the fat—and the Oreos, and anything else that wasn't tied down—about how we were going to get ourselves back into shape, since she also looked like a normal middle-aged woman who had had a bunch of kids. She came over to tell me about the anniversary present her husband had given her. He was taking her to San Francisco to an exercise physiologist who was teaching a fancy breathing exercise she called "the Rolls-Royce of exercise" and who charged $1,500 for ten one-on-one classes. She claimed the technique would produce inch loss overnight and increase energy and vibrancy, all without dieting. "There's a sucker born every minute," I told my neighbor.

I may have lost my appetite but I was still forced to eat those words when I saw my neighbor three weeks later when she came back from San Francisco. Not only had she gone down two dress sizes, but her entire countenance and energy level was different. Though, to my logical mind, the thought of standing still and breathing and losing inches a week seemed bizarre, I was a desperate woman rapidly approaching a size 16. I was like someone who had a terminal illness and was told she could be healed if she packed her body with mud and ran around in a circle backwards—I was willing to try anything, and desperate times called for desperate measures. And all it took was that somebody I personally knew and could see with my own two eyes had gotten results.

So, in what was to be my last-ditch effort to get myself in shape, I decided to take the classes even though my husband, who was not making big money because he had not as yet branched out on his own, jokingly told me that if I spent our hard-earned dollars on this, we were through. Great, a loophole! I thought. But I didn't care how much effort it took, how much money it cost, or what I had to do. It had worked for my neighbor and I felt it could work for me. In any case, I was willing to try. To a point.

A Breath of Fresh Air

I went to San Francisco and enrolled in the program. I can remember very vividly walking into a big room, like a hotel conference room, with all these chairs set up theater style. I took a seat in the back, where all the older and larger women seemed to be sitting, while the younger, thinner women sat in the front. I had my arms folded, ready to do battle, daring anyone to convince me that this really was going to work. I'm like a lot of people: I'm serious when I say I'm going to do something, but the second I get there, I'm ready to go home. Forget that this was California; I lived in the state of doubt. As that feeling washed over me, the only thing keeping me in that chair was the image of my now slender, vibrant, energetic neighbor who currently was everything I wanted to be.

I don't know what I expected, but I know what I didn't—the twentysomething young thing who looked like she took her meals out of a birdfeeder who came strolling out of a side room to stand at the head of the class. "Who the heck is that?" I said to the woman next to me. "She's an exercise physiologist," she replied. Trust me, there's nothing more aggravating than hearing a sweet young thing who looks like she has the appetite and metabolism of a sparrow trying to tell overweight, unfit women who have had kids how their butts can be like this and their thighs can be like that and their stomachs, faces, and arms can look like so. I wondered what this person could possibly know about me, my kids, my fat, and my sag. So, possessing the big mouth that I do, I decided to find out.

"How many kids do you have?" I hollered out from the back row. "I don't have any," the exercise physiologist sheepishly replied. To which I responded out loud, "Well, then, I'm done listening." Still, desperation and the words inside my head, "This worked for my friend," kept me tied to that chair and glued to what she was saying in a way that ropes and Elmer's couldn't have done half as well. I still didn't like her—she was so committed, convincing, and determined about this program—but ultimately, I realized that I hated my body and the way I felt more than I hated her. So, with arms folded in resistance the entire time, and with a countenance that was punishing this physiologist by making it known that I was seemingly listening with only half an ear, I stayed. And I got my first lesson on the importance of aerobic breathing.

For me, it turned out to be an exercise in the power of negative thinking—you know, imagine the worst and good things happen in spite of you. I kept telling myself that the program wasn't going to work and I was kind of hoping and praying it wasn't going to work so that I could be right. (I think we're all afraid to *really* believe that something out there is going to do the trick.) The funny part was that, as I learned how to do the program, I knew in my heart of hearts that it was going to do what I wanted it to do. I saw results after day one in my energy level. At that point, I said to myself, I don't care if I don't lose any inches or weight, I feel better and that has to be worth something. The first few days, I honestly didn't see any change in my body, but my stress level went down even more as my energy level went up. After seven days, I began to see a little difference in the mirror. But when I had myself measured, I discovered I had lost 10½ inches the first week! Of course, it's kind of "the watched pot never boils theory"—10½ inches spread out over your midsection (a half an inch here, an inch there, two inches here) and your arms is hard for you to see because you look at yourself every day. But when I went home after that week, people were beginning to say, "Gee, you look good. Whatcha doing, Greer?"

I figured I wasn't going to say anything and just wait and see how long it would take to have dramatic results. But there was no disputing that my energy continued to build every day and that I found myself less and less on the couch watching TV and more and more interested in going out, in keeping the house up, and in living life instead of just vegging around and being despondent. I was finally able to get off the antidepressants. My kids—then infant, seven, and seventeen—found me much happier and calmer to be around. And I finally had something to look forward to.

With three kids, however, I was unable to spare the hour and a half each day that the program took. So I did it for forty-five minutes a day instead, doing the exercises for the parts of my body that needed them the most. Then I even began shaving time off of that. In the end, I did the program for thirty-five minutes a day religiously for four months; plus, if I found myself getting tired at night, I would go into the bathroom and do ten more of the breaths and, boom, I'd be ready for the rest of the night. Again, it's a process: Your body isn't used to carrying so much oxygen and you're used to being tired, so you may alternate between being energetic and tired until it balances out. But at the end of three months, I was down to a size 4–6, plus I felt terrific.

At the end of five months, now busy, on the go, and feeling good, I decided to experiment and quit the program for three weeks or so. It didn't take long for me to remember why I had done the exercises to begin with, as I slipped back into feeling the awful way I had in the past, all the while watching myself begin to spread once more. As my clothes started getting tighter around the waist, I thought, No thanks. I wasn't going back to that size 14–16, which would have been easy to do because the inches creep up on you without your even realizing how fast it happens. I went back on the program and have been doing it ever since.

Actually, I thought it was the most wonderful thing in the world that I was able to lose fat and eat normally. After being down that long road to trying to get in shape, I proclaimed that I was never, never, ever going to diet again. To me, eating is one of the joys of living, and I refused to punish myself day after day by telling myself I couldn't have this and I couldn't have that. So I went on my merry way and ate exactly what I wanted to eat, as long as I could lift it with a fork. Back then I didn't know what healthy eating was. I figured as long as I wasn't eating pork and beans, I was okay. I'd prepare breakfast for my family and eat with them. Then, for lunch, I'd have maybe a sandwich, a salad, and a bowl of soup. In the evening, I'd fix dinner for my husband and kids and we'd all sit down and eat. I didn't sacrifice—I'm telling you the truth.

Of course, I wasn't on a steady diet of fried chicken and Twinkies either. But as a result of doing my exercises each day, my metabolism sped up and I was able to process my food faster and differently. The thing about this exercise is that it naturally reduces your appetite; it's not something you consciously do. But I could eat what I wanted and not gain weight, be firm, and have energy all at the same time. Is that the cat's pajamas or what? I was so happy I felt as if

I was in outer space. The best part was that I was taking up very little room.

I did keep asking myself how this technique could possibly work. Frankly, at the time I was completely ignorant of the facts. The exercise physiologist who taught it to me didn't understand it either, so she couldn't explain why and how this method produced results. But the truth was, I didn't give a rip how it worked. All I knew was that I had taken ten classes in five days, then come home and did the program on my own, and within three months I went from a size 14–16 to a size 4–6, where I remain today. Not only that, but, for the first time in years I felt vibrant. Vibrancy is the key to everything, particularly to the quality of life.

What was so gratifying was that I couldn't walk down the street without someone approaching me to ask me what I had done to get so slim and improve my overall appearance so much. (And, yes, the sidewalks of Salt Lake City had finally been separated from my butt in this wonderful nonsurgical procedure.) When I told people I had done a breathing exercise, many displayed the same skepticism I had initially felt, and they snickered and walked off whispering, "Yeah, she probably starved herself." But a lot wanted me to teach them. Unfortunately, I wasn't qualified to do so.

I then went back to the physiologist who had taught me the program and told her, "Look, you need to bring this to the general public because this is something that could benefit the housewife, the schoolteacher, the construction worker. Everybody out there is desperate and needs help and there's nothing out there—I know because there was nothing for me until this." She told me that she couldn't reduce the price, repeating again that it was "the Rolls-Royce of exercise" and that it was for the elite, the rich, the fa-mous.

What a selfish attitude, I thought. Something that can really change the quality of someone's life should be available to all. Average American women don't take limos; they need a more affordable means to get around. There had to be a way to streamline this method into a shorter and more doable program—the one the physiologist had taught me was ninety minutes long and consisted of positions and exercises it seemed to me you practically had to be an Olympic-level gymnast to accomplish. I just had to bring it to the thousands of women and men everywhere who needed it, at a price that wouldn't leave a hole in their wallets. I said to the physiologist, "I know nothing because I'm just a housewife with no education or trade, but I'm going to make it my business to find out how and why this breathing program works and when I do, I'm going to take it to the general public." I had found my mission.

The Birth of BodyFlex

With that, I began what turned into four and a half years of research into this breathing technique. I used my own time and all my money to fly all over the country and meet with specialists in every field of medicine to gather data and understand why and how the program worked so that I could educate my potential clients. Unlike the person who had taught me, I didn't want to just fly by the seat of my pants. In the process, I learned more physiology than some doctors. I was not only excited to learn how and why this technique burns fat but also the other health benefits it provides.

I'm just like the average person: I don't like exercising and I like to eat. I am also a believer in taking the path of least resistance, in taking something complicated and making it simple. I wanted my exercise program to fit into a time frame that would give people no excuse not to exercise. I knew my success rate with my customers was going to be extremely low if I kept the program at an hour and a half—they were going to tell me that they didn't have that amount of time to work out. But I felt it would be awfully hard for them to look me in the eye and tell me they didn't have fifteen minutes . . . especially when I would be telling them that the average participant would lose 4 to 14 inches in their midsection alone the first week if they did the program for just fifteen minutes a day. So I incorporated very simple isometric and isotonic positions that would be extremely effective in fifteen minutes a day if the breathing was done right. My research and testing confirmed that, using these positions in conjunction with the breathing, participants could reap the maximum benefits in that time frame as opposed to an hour and a half a day.

What I had learned through my research, and as I'll explain in greater detail in Chapter 3, was that if you put stress on a particular area of the body, as you do with these positions, you create a need for more blood to that area. Oxygen is carried to the areas of the body through the blood, and oxygen burns fat while isometric and isotonic positions tone muscle. The secret to my program is to do both simultaneously. We don't want to just drop twenty pounds, we want to lose body fat and inches at the same time so that we become firm and fit. We want our thighs not to shake when we walk, our triceps not to swing when we wave, and our stomach not to flop on the bed on its own when we lie down on our side.

In 1985, I was living in Houston, Texas, by this time a divorced mother of three (I finally had to drop-kick the doctor) who often didn't have enough money for groceries. Even in Houston, people were always coming up to me and asking me how I got and stayed so slim. Feeling that I had learned enough about the breathing method to teach my neighbors and friends, and having streamlined the program down to fifteen minutes with isometric and isotonic positions that just about everyone could do, or could at least be adapted to everyone, I went to work. I typed up an advertisement on recipe cards and put the cards on bulletin boards in grocery stores and in Laundromats. My slogan was "A face lift, a tummy tuck, a total body lift in less than fifteen minutes a day, without surgery or dieting. Average person loses 4 to 14 inches the first week."

The first week I got one or two calls; the second week, four; the third week, ten—and it just kept building. Soon I was getting calls from companies to give a free talk to their employees, after which they all wanted to take the class. I was teaching every day, charging $75 a person. Then I got a call from a woman who was going to be in a beauty pageant in forty-five days. She said that if I could get her down from her size 12–14 to a size 6 by then, she would get me a job at one of the largest health club chains in Texas. Well, she made it and so did I. I taught two to three classes a day in those clubs. Houston is the largest city in Texas, so the news that I had created an affordable program that really worked traveled fast. I was invited to be the keynote speaker for the Commerce Club and the Chamber of Commerce and at meetings for big corporations like Southwestern Bell, who had two thousand people present at a luncheon, after which the first question was "When can we do it?" "All of you?" I inquired. I had to break up the group into several different classes, teaching one class a day.

Greer in High Gear

After busting my butt and teaching classes for years, never changing my $75-a-person fee, I came to the conclusion that I needed a way to reach the masses. While I did hire some of my best students to teach various classes for me, no one knows the program like the person who developed it, and I'd often have to end up reteaching some of the people they had taught. So, in 1990, after moving back to Utah for family reasons, I made my first video, a simple instructional one showing people the BodyFlex technique. The next question was how to market it.

By this time, I had saved up enough money not only to pay for the video but to make an infomercial done without using any investors as well as pay for my own airtime. I hired a production company to do the infomercial and wrote the script for it myself. Rather than hire a media buyer to purchase the airtime for me, I researched the market and bought my own, buying superstations all over the country from KTLA in Los Angeles to WGN in Chicago. To take the orders, I used the services of Matrix, the largest 1-800 inbound company in the world.

All the professionals had told me that I had to be more polished in the infomercial; I couldn't just look into the camera and talk to the general public like I was an ordinary housewife. I told them that it was my money and my business and I would talk to my prospective clients without any fancy words, just with a down-home presentation. Believability is the key to success in this business. I think we're all fed up with young hardbodies telling us how to bounce back from a place they've never been. Who better to tell ordinary men and women how to get into shape than one of their own? I tell the truth, which is why BodyFlex is so successful. My infomercial lasted one year, during which time I sold 350,000 videos.

I stopped teaching classes two years ago after moving to Las Vegas, and in 1996, I began my foray into the Home Shopping Network and QVC. I can never forget that it is the everyday woman and man who are going through the same pain I went through as an overweight, unhappy person. That is the focal point of my mission. We're all the same. No matter how much money you have, what you look like, or what station you are in life, we're all the same inside. We all want the same things. The biggest thrill I get is when I go on a show to talk about BodyFlex and folks who've done the program call in and tell me how it's changed their lives. I listen to how happy they are and I feel so grateful that my program could make a difference in their health and vitality. I think each one of us has a contribution to make, and I'm glad I found something that finally works that I can bring to my fellow woman and man.

And now, I'd like to share my BodyFlex program with you. I hope it brings you as much joy and vitality as it's brought me.

2.

Stop Using That Awful F Word

*T*here is just no nice way to say the word *fat*. Heavy . . . overweight . . . pleasantly plump . . . zaftig—they all have the same derogatory connotation. Here we are, down in the trenches doing all we can, and we remain fat and frustrated. Overweight and obesity are at an all-time high in this country. It is estimated that currently the vast majority of the population is overweight and/or out of shape and 35 percent of the American populace is clinically obese (that is, more than 20 percent above the ideal weight for their height).

How does weight creep up on us the way it does? If we've been pigging out, we can understand why the needle on the scale goes up, but for most of us, the weight gain is a mystery. We do the same old thing, day after day, then, all of sudden, we start putting on pounds. We're not doing anything differently, but we can't get rid of them. And we don't know what to do because we haven't made any changes in our lives and we don't understand what's happening to us.

So we run to the doctor thinking we have a thyroid problem, and the doctor looks at us and says, "What's happening is that you're getting a little older and your metabolism is slowing down a little bit." He or she recommends exercise because we need to jump-start our metabolism and try to boost it back up to what it used to be so that we can process our food faster, burn our calories faster, and be able to eat more and weigh less. The doctor may encourage us to do aerobic exercise, but what he or she may not explain is that the *only* way to speed up metabolism is through aerobic breathing.

The best part is that you don't have to jump, hop, and run to become aerobic. The word *aerobic* means increasing oxygen to the body through breathing. And the element that burns fat in the body is oxygen. So you see, being aerobic has absolutely nothing to do with movement. You can become aerobic standing still, sitting still, even lying down if you know how to breathe aerobically. In fact, you can become aerobic much more easily through breathing than you can through movement. Because the movement is just designed to stress your body to get you to . . . guess what? Right! Breathe more deeply, thereby increasing oxygen to the body to make you become aerobic to . . . guess what? Right again! Burn fat. So you can either do a whole lot of movement to get yourself to breathe more deeply, or you can learn to breathe more efficiently and aerobically—and that's what BodyFlex is all about.

T*he Difference Between Fat and Flab*

But if you really want to look and feel good, just losing weight or excess body fat is not enough. People are forever coming up to me and saying, "Can you help me drop twenty pounds?" Well, yeah, I can help you drop twenty pounds. But is that what you really want? I've talked to many disappointed people who have lost the weight they've wanted to lose and have told me that they look worse than they did before. Why? Because their thighs are still lumpy, their stomachs are still poochy, and their butts are still sagging. And they haven't been able to drop their dress or suit size. That's because they haven't tightened the soft or untoned muscle, which is that other nasty F word, the big four-letter F word: "flab"—you know, sagging skin, arms that keep waving long after you've stopped, thighs that keep going and going and going way after you've stopped moving. In other words, losing weight and being in shape are two entirely different things. Lose the fat in the areas you want to and tighten these areas up at the same time and you'll get the results you're looking for.

The ultimate goal of BodyFlex is not weight loss; it's toning and shaping and high energy. I have had clients who have gone down two dress sizes yet never lost a pound. They simply became smaller by tightening up the untoned muscle. I have worked with thousands of people who think they are grossly overweight and they drop down a couple of dress sizes and lose two or three pounds and look as if they've lost fifty pounds and look fabulous. That's because they had excess flab on their bodies, not excess weight. And most people can't tell the difference between the two. When someone has a large thigh, for example, she may think it's fat, but it's really flab—untoned muscle.

What happens to people who are really heavy and then lose a lot of weight is this: When they are fat, their skin is rather tight. As they start losing body fat, the skin starts to sag because it loses its elasticity. The skin is like a rubber band. Stretch it out and it's taut and then release it and it's flaccid. Or think of it this way: When you blow up a balloon to its maximum, that balloon is full and firm and tight. But if you let half the air out of the balloon, what happens? The film on the outside becomes soft and loose and saggy. When you deplete what's inside that balloon, the outer surface just relaxes.

As I said before, flab is soft or untoned muscle. Like the balloon, when the skin is filled with fat, it is nice and firm and tight. When you start burning that excess body fat and you don't tighten the muscle simultaneously, you have untoned muscle, loose skin, saggy flabby inner thighs, outer thighs, arms, stomach, and rear end.

Luckily, there can be a happy ending to the saga of "The Good, the Flab, and the Ugly." BodyFlex burns excess body fat (by increasing oxygen to the system, you can utilize or burn eighteen times more fat in your cells than by doing exercise that isn't aerobic) and tones muscle simultaneously with a combination of aerobic breathing and isometric, isotonic, and stretch positions. In other words, you won't lose twenty pounds and still have a poochy stomach and swinging thighs. The end result is inch loss. Results vary, but in my direct observation the inch loss of the average participant on this program is 4 to 14 inches in the midsection—the stomach, hips, thighs, and lower and upper abs—the first week. And what inch loss produces is a tight, trim body best described by that nice F word: "fit." And a fit body is the ticket to good health.

Throw Away Your Scale

I tell people on the BodyFlex program, "Throw that scale away." I don't care what people weigh. I'm trying to get people out of thinking, "If I lose ten pounds or I lose twenty pounds, I'll be where I want to be," because it may not be at all where they want to be. We are geared in this country to weight loss, weight loss, weight loss. And people fling themselves into a miserable cycle of calorie deprivation and binging, followed by more dieting. Food has nothing to do with this program; in other words, you don't have to diet. In terms of appearance, all we care about at BodyFlex are two things: how we look and what size we are. I ask my clients, "Do you want to be a size 8 if you're a size 12? Do you want to go from a size 14 to a size 10? If your waist is twenty-seven inches, do you want it to be twenty-three inches? What results do you want?" It's a totally different way of looking at exercise.

Though this program is not about weight, in the process of doing BodyFlex, you *will* burn excess body fat. And most women have excess body fat because of the way fat is naturally deposited on their bodies and the way hormones keep it there. Those hormones also cause 85 percent of women to have cellulite, which is deposits of fat stored with a lot of metabolic waste (chemicals from food and food by-products). BodyFlex also helps breaks down cellulite.

But, with this program, we focus on inches, because fighting flab is where it's at. When you turn flab into muscle, you lose inches. The key is that our bodies know where they are supposed to be weightwise. And people can be lulled into a false sense of looking good if they focus on pound loss. I am 5 feet 10 inches tall and weigh 151 pounds, and if you never saw me, you might think I'm fat. After all, those supermodels who are my height weigh 115 or 120 pounds. Surprise! I am a size 4–6. In fact, I went from a size 14–16 to a size 4–6 on this program and only lost forty-five pounds.

We all know one thing about fitness: You have to become aerobic to burn body fat. *And the aerobic part of all exercise is in the breathing.* That is the backbone of all exercise. The problem with most people is that they are thirty pounds overweight to begin with, then they go to the gym and say that they are going to start working out and tighten those flabby arms, legs, and other body parts. But when they work out and start the ab rolling, crunching, and butt blasting, they don't become aerobic enough to burn the fat off their bodies, so what they end up doing is building muscle under the existing layers of fat, of which there are several. That produces results opposite to what most of us want—they get bigger rather than smaller, achieving nothing more than a bulky body.

Have you ever heard people say, "I'm not getting on a stair stepper because all I'll get is a big butt?" If you understand the philosophy of exercise, you can understand why this happens. You're stepping, stepping, stepping up and down, but not getting aerobic enough to burn the fat. So what you are doing is building those muscles all right, right in your behind, because you are putting stress on the gluteus maximus; the fat stays there because you aren't burning it off. So again, you are building muscle under existing fat.

Do you want to be able to see the curves of the muscles in your legs, arms, and back? The only way to do that is to reduce the amount of body fat you're carrying around and simultaneously tone the muscle underneath so that you can see the definition, or muscle tone, that's being developed. The idea is to *tone* muscle, by the way, not *build* muscle. When you look at a bodybuilder, what you see is a big middle, big arms, big legs, big chest. He uses weights to build muscle. Now watch him walk. You'll notice that he has little flexibility; he moves kind of like a refrigerator.

That's because he has shortened and bulked up the muscle; that's where he gets his big muscles.

What we do at BodyFlex is the opposite—we elongate muscle. We stretch, lean, and breathe so that we tone muscle and have more flexibility because we know that range of motion is so critical as we get older. We know that bodybuilders have a difficult time because they are prone to injury due to their lack of flexibility and range of motion. With BodyFlex, we end up being able to bend and stretch and reach and move and do the things we need to do as we're getting older. We want a livable lifestyle and that means being able to stay on our feet and move around for as long as possible.

What Are You Running, Hopping, and Jumping For, Anyway?

In my opinion, the most misunderstood notion people have is about what aerobic exercise is. I've asked people from all over the world what they think it is. They tell me it's about running, moving, getting your arms and legs going, and so on. Then I ask them, "Why are you doing it?" And they give me all sorts of answers: "To get my heart rate up." "To burn calories." "To make myself sweat." "To build up my cardiovascular system." I keep pressing them: "Why do you want to get your heart rate up? Why do you need to sweat? Why do you want to build up your cardiovascular system?" They don't know how to answer those questions, because they don't understand how it all fits together logically.

The answer is simple: *You do aerobic exercise to increase the amount of oxygen delivered to the cells of your body.* All exercise works on exactly the same principle: You have to increase oxygen in the blood and then direct the oxygenated blood to the areas you want it to affect, giving the working muscle group the ability to utilize the oxygen you deliver to it. Whether lifting weights, riding a bike, or whatever, this is how it works—any time you put a stress or a stretch on a particular area of the body, what you do is create a need for more blood to that area. Blood is the transportation system for oxygen and oxygen is the fat-burning ingredient the body needs in order to burn the excess fat we're carrying around. So what we need to do is increase oxygen to the body so that we can have more fat-burning ability.

Regular exercise, as long as it's stressing a part of the body, will build muscle but it doesn't necessarily burn fat. That's because you're working out anaerobically, which means that you're not breathing deeply enough to supply oxygen to the working muscles. What you're doing instead is using the glucose, or blood sugar, in a localized area of your body for energy. Have you ever gotten the shakes after doing regular exercise, or gotten so hungry right afterward that you wanted to eat everything and anything? That's because you lowered your blood sugar level and your body is trying to get it back up. The point is that when you want to lose excess body fat, you have to use that fat for energy instead of sugar. And the only way you can use the fat is if you get a lot of oxygen into the blood to burn it and supply it to the working muscles. That can only be done by aerobic breathing.

Everyone has fat cells; we can never get rid of them (unless we get them sucked out through liposuction). The idea is to keep them depleted. In an effort to tell you everything you always wanted to know about fat and were afraid to ask, I'll give you a few scientific facts about fat. Let's say you start out at a certain weight and you have a hundred fat cells. As you gain more and more weight over a certain period of time, you'll reach a point where those fat cells get fat. While it's okay to lose weight, what you really want to do is lower your percentage of body fat, which is measured as the difference between muscle and fat in your body. The muscle is toned through exercise, getting the calories (energy) to do so from the fat, which is the storage place in the body for calories. The fat also releases the free fatty acids and the glycerol needed to tone muscle. Thus, you are burning fat to enhance the muscle. It is like a balancing act. And BodyFlex works in two ways: providing spot muscle development, hence toning, in an aerobic state, meaning that it both builds a great foundation for muscle and increases metabolism through breathing to burn fat.

Fit, Not Fat

Can you be fit and fat at the same time? Not to my way of thinking. It has been medically proven many times over that too much body fat is at the root of too many illnesses. Five years ago, the average dress size of the American woman was a size 12. Well, we've certainly come a long way (make that a wide way), baby, because today the average dress size is a size 14. That's too big. The surgeon general has said that one-third of the American people are clinically obese. And the saddest thing is that the other two-thirds are headed in the same direction.

So fitness is more than lack of excess body fat and

good muscle tone. Being fit also means that your choles-terol, triglycerides, blood pressure, heart rate, and the like are all where they're supposed to be and that you are in shape cardiovascularly. That means that you are working the lungs, heart, and the muscles around them, strength-ening them and providing optimum circulation throughout the body. Every cell must have adequate oxygen. Fitness has to be inside and out. What we need is something that's a total package for the entire body, both inside and out. That's BodyFlex.

Most of us don't want to admit that we're in bad shape cardiovascularly. So I'm going to give you this simple little test. Start at the bottom of a flight of stairs and take the stairs up, two at a time. I guarantee that you'll be so winded by the time you reach the top that you won't know what hit you. Then, after you've done deep diaphragmatic breathing with BodyFlex for a few weeks, try this test again. You'll find you'll be able to head up those stairs two at a time, four or five times, and you won't even be winded. That means that you're in a heck of a lot better cardiovascular shape than you used to be. That's one of the first things people notice on this program. And you'll have learned an important lesson: You don't have to run, jump, and hop around to build up your cardiovascular system; you just have to learn how to breathe more aerobically. *It's the breathing, not the moving.*

Most people don't understand what fitness is. They are no different from the way I was. Do you know that all those years I was doing this and that and the other thing, I didn't even know why I was exercising? Someone told me to do this and someone else told me I needed to do that, but I had no clue as to why I was doing any of it. If someone told me it was going to work, I just did it.

I believe that if people truly understood how exercise works, they wouldn't jump to try the latest craze on the market out of desperation. If somebody tells them that if they stand on their heads and line BBs up in a row that they'll lose 10 inches, it's, "Hey, count me in." They waste a lot of time because they just don't understand the dynamics of exercise and how it works. Or what it really means to be fit.

Total fitness, in my book, is looking as good as you possibly can and having the vibrancy you've always wanted. The common denominator among all healthy people is energy and a zest for life, while the common denominator among all sick people is a lack of energy and dullness. Know this for sure: When you have energy and feel good, it can almost be guaranteed that you are healthy and fit on the inside.

To get on the right path to fitness, you need to change your mind-set. You're not looking for the exercise that makes you sweat the most, burn the most calories, move around the most, or pant the hardest. You want the exercise that will get the most fat-burning oxygen to your cells. You don't need to work harder, you need to breathe more efficiently.

The more you understand how BodyFlex works, the more motivated I think you'll be to try it and stay with it. In the next chapter, I'll tell you more about why and how deep breathing can make a huge difference in the quality of your life.

3.

Here's the Skinny on Oxygen

I call oxygen "the non-medical miracle." All over the world now, people are catching on to what this element can do. Oxygen therapies are becoming so popular that there are oxygen bars, oxygen creams, oxygen pep-ups, and more. That's because more oxygen can help everything from overweight to low energy to poor health. One of the things I find very interesting is that *Prevention Magazine's* 1997 Best Home Remedies claims that the best solution for headaches, depression, cellulite, dropped bladder, and a multitude of other problems is deep breathing. Does oxygenation through deep breathing live up to all these claims and more? You bet it does. I am telling you that you can have a healthier lifestyle, a more powerful immune system, and a leaner body . . . simply by breathing.

Everybody says, when they first hear about it, "This is the craziest thing I've ever heard." We all make fun of things we don't understand. I've already told you the basis of BodyFlex—an accelerated aerobic breathing technique that oxygenates the system. That means it delivers vital oxygen to the body, delivering it to the blood, which, in turn, delivers it to our cells.

If you still don't understand the importance of oxygenation, listen to Paul Bragg, author of *Super Power Breathing for Super Energy* and also the person who developed the first health food store in this country in the late

1930s. As he says in his book, we are slowly committing sui-
cide in this country because of the way we live and breathe.
He claims that we are actually suffocating.

According to Bragg, shallow breathing starves the
body of vital oxygen and causes premature aging. Bragg
notes that oxygen-starved people go to bed tired and wake
up tired. They suffer from headaches, constipation, indiges-
tion, muscular aches and pains, stiff joints, aching backs
and feet, aching teeth and sore receding gums, poor eye-
sight, poor hearing, loss of memory, sore throats, and respiratory ailments such as bronchitis, asthma, sinus infections,
and emphysema. He maintains that these miseries and loss
of healthy bodily functions plague these people early in life
and take them to an early grave.

Not only do we breathe shallowly (I'll discuss this in
detail in the next chapter), but we are suffering from what
might be called a double whammy. Two hundred years ago,
our air was composed of 38 percent oxygen and 1 percent
carbon dioxide. Today, because of pollution and other factors, it is 19 percent oxygen and 25 percent carbon dioxide.
(Everyone thinks that the oxygen in the air comes from the
trees and the forests. But the truth is that 90 percent of it
comes from the sea, from sealife, algae, etc., only 10 percent comes from the forests.) Not only do people in Western cultures breathe shallowly, barely using *one-fifth* of the
lungs' capacity to increase oxygen flow to their bodies, but,
on top of everything else, there is much less oxygen in the
air to breathe.

According to Norman McVea, M.D., Ph.D., in *Wellness Lifestyle* magazine, besides pollution, other reasons for
oxygen depletion are planetary deforestation, chlorinated
water, devitalized soil, processed foods, chemical pollu-

tants, automobile emissions, and electronic smog, not to mention problems within our own bodies: stress; bacterial, viral, and fungal infections; clogged colons; lack of exercise; and poor dietary, posture, and breathing habits.

Dr. McVea explains the importance of oxygen this way: "More than anything else, good health and well-being is dependent on the maximum production, maintenance and flow of energy, which is produced by oxygen.

"Oxygen contributes to proper metabolic function, better circulation, assimilation, digestion and elimination," McVea continues. "It helps purify the blood, keeping it free from cellular build-up. Sufficient oxygen gives the body a chance to rebuild itself and strengthen its immune system, our natural defense against disease. . . . It also has a calming and energizing effect on the nervous system. Oxidation is the key to life."

We also know that over 90 percent of the body's energy is produced by oxygen, and that the more oxygen we have in our system, the more we produce. That's more important than ever before because of our general deficiency of oxygen intake. Our ability to think, feel, and act comes from the energy created by oxygen. Most of us are tired because we simply don't have enough oxygen in our systems.

In a recent article in the *Journal of Longevity* entitled "Oxygen Decrease Leading to Worldwide Increase in Disease," the author, Dr. Philip C. Stavish, concurs that we are slowly suffocating from lack of oxygen and that oxygen deficiency causes everything from a feeling of uneasiness to full-blown illness. He states that oxygen depletion—not global warming—is the real danger facing mankind and that we are at a near-crisis point concerning the oxygen in our air and in our cells.

"Oxygen deficiency results in a weakened immune system, which can lead to viral problems, damaged cell growths, toxic buildup in the blood, and premature aging—among other ailments," Dr. Stavish notes.

Moreover, Stavish cites the alarming statistic that there has been a 50 percent decrease in the oxygen in the air—from 38 percent down to 19 to 21 percent—and says that what is disturbing researchers is that the human body was originally designed to operate with a 50 percent stronger concentration of oxygen in the atmosphere.

According to Stavish, scientists have measured oxygen levels as low as 12 to 15 percent.

Oxygen is essential for cell growth and regeneration. Oxygen also provides the fat-burning ingredient for the body. So, BodyFlex has two purposes: (1) to increase oxygen flow and deliver it to the bloodstream so that we are able to burn more body fat, and (2) to give us a healthier body along with it. We need to get more oxygen to our cells so that we can boost our energy level and have more vibrancy. And vibrancy is tantamount to good health.

O*xygen Burns Fat*

In the 1980s I asked a professor at Baylor University in Texas to explain how BodyFlex works. He said that anything that burns is considered a fuel. Fuels are usually divided into categories based upon their ease of combustion, or "burnability." In the body, the highest grade fuel—in terms of combustion—is fat, or lipids. The additional oxygen brought into the body through BodyFlex helps oxidize, or burn, that high-grade fuel. Breaking down these lipids means reducing fat in the areas where the most fat has collected.

As the professor explained, as you continue the BodyFlex breathing, you bring more oxygen into the body, which the body now has to manage. It's like bringing a lot of new automobiles into a city. The city managers begin to build new expressways and roadways to handle the additional traffic. This is accomplished in the body by generating new arteries, veins, and capillaries to handle the additional oxygen supply. As the lipids are burned off, the oxygen continues to interact with other components of the body, generating healthier and stronger muscles, and nerve, organ, and skin tissue as well, thereby developing muscle tone, strength, endurance, and vigor.

If you lack energy, it may be the result of the internal sensory control network's monitoring of oxygen levels in the blood. When levels are low, your body can respond by conserving its energy by reducing its output. This translates into a lowered drive and less physical activity. In short, you feel run down. When the blood oxygen levels are increased through aerobic activity such as BodyFlex, the sensory control network sends a message to allow more energy output, resulting in increased drive, vitality, and capability.

O*xygen, Stress, and the Immune System*

There are already scores of medical practitioners who recognize the value of deep breathing and the list is growing. For example, world-renowned cardiologist Dr. Dean Ornish says in his book *Dr. Dean Ornish's Program for Reversing Heart Disease* that deep breathing is the best stress reducer known to man. Stress can kill you and anything you can do to de-stress your life can help lengthen your life. The word from the medical community has spread. It's no surprise that all the leading motivational speakers and trainers teach deep breathing as a form of relaxation and as a stress eliminator. Tony Robbins even has a whole chapter on breathing in his book *Unlimited Power.*

Think about the last time you got sick. It was probably at a time when you were at a high point of stress. It has been proven that stress has a direct impact on the immune system. It's like a teeter-totter. When your stress level is up, your immune system is down; when your stress level is down, your immune system is up. Stress is a major plague in this country. If we can reduce our stress through deep breathing, we can help boost our immune systems.

We need to keep our immune systems strong so we can fight off sickness. The immune system is our number-one line of defense against the viruses, bacteria, and other invaders that make us ill, causing everything from minor colds and flus to some major illnesses.

Doctors have long been recommending exercise for anyone who gets a lot of colds and such. What they really want their patients to do is to increase their breathing to increase the oxygen levels in the blood to strengthen our immune systems so that viruses and bacteria can't survive. Again, you don't need a brisk jog to raise your oxygen levels; you can do it with deep breathing. I can personally testify to the benefits of deep breathing to strengthen the immune system: I haven't had a cold in ten years.

"Greer has a certain technique that she borrowed from the ancient cultures to keep one's immune system primed for this society," states Burton Goldberg, author of *Alternative Medicine: The Definitive Guide,* in an interview with me and my cowriter. "BodyFlex is one of the greatest catalysts to keeping the immune system peaked. In fact, BodyFlex is a total package for total health and is one of the incredibly inexpensive things you can do for yourself to control your own destiny. I do it myself for well-being, relaxation, tension reduction, and for overall health. You can't argue with success and clinically it works—millions of people are getting results. You can use the knowledge on the pages of this book to get well and stay well."

"Oxygen gets rid of toxicity," concurs Alec Borsenko, a naturopath, author, and expert on colon health whom my cowriter and I interviewed. "Bacteria, viruses, and parasites are destroyed in the presence of oxygen—especially cancer. BodyFlex is the best technique on the market for getting oxygen into your system. It gets you aerobic five times faster than running—if you ran for an hour, you would burn 700 calories; if you did Jazzercise for an hour, you would burn 250 calories; if you did BodyFlex for an hour, you would burn 3,500 calories."

Oxygen and Chronic Diseases

What happens when you do a system like BodyFlex, in which you oxygenate the blood day after day, is that you increase the amount of oxygen to the blood. It will help keep you in a healthy state. That's why many people who have Epstein-Barr virus, otherwise known as chronic fatigue syndrome, have had such a great response to this exercise. Many experts believe that these people are tired all the time, are very weak all the time, and end up getting sick all the time because there is a lack of oxygen to the system. They can't get well because they are shallow, tidal breathers (see the next chapter) to begin with, and because they are so weak, they breathe even more shallowly. The theory is that the lack of oxygen to the body keeps the virus in the system and allows it to reproduce. Oxygenation could be the answer. In fact, there is a book on the market called *Chronic Fatigue and Other Illnesses* touting deep breathing exercises as a remedy for chronic fatigue syndrome. I have hundreds of clients with chronic fatigue syndrome who tell me their conditions have dramatically improved since they began BodyFlex.

Noted medical researcher/scientist/Ph.D., author, and lecturer Dr. Daniel Mowrey, in his book *Fat Management: The Thermogenic Factor,* singles out the BodyFlex program in his discussion of the benefits of deep breathing because it has the advantage of not raising the body's core temperature very much and because it definitely produces fat loss and inch loss. During normal exercise, when you are jumping and running and working the muscles really hard, your body's core temperature increases, which can promote muscle degeneration in some people. That's why those suffering from diseases like multiple sclerosis have to be very careful about exercise, because raising their body's core temperature can cause further degeneration. People with MS can do BodyFlex—with their doctor's go-ahead— because it doesn't contribute to the deterioration of their condition. For a well person, the fact that the body's core temperature doesn't rise simply means that it's an easier, more effective, and healthier way to exercise.

World-famous immunologist and medical researcher Dr. Sheldon Hendler has written several books. In his latest, *The Oxygen Breakthrough,* he writes: "You can rid your body of chronic illness by deep breathing exercises." His book describes one case study after another attesting to the fact that the delivery of oxygen to the blood will help detoxify the system and keep viruses and bacteria at a minimum because they cannot reproduce in the blood when there is ample oxygen present. That evidence alone should make everyone sit up and take notice of what a powerful impact their breathing has on their health.

Oxygen, Anxiety, and Depression

Oxygenation can also help reduce anxiety and depression, which are also at the root of so much physical disease. Julian Whittaker, the author of the largest medical newsletter in North America, writes in his publication: "A runner may be arrogant, may be smug, may be snotty, but he'll never be depressed."

Some of you reading this book may be able to identify with the following scenario: You're depressed, you're crying and you don't know why, you're tired, you're dragging around, you don't know what's wrong but you know you have no interest in anything. The first thing a doctor will tell you is to get on an exercise program—walk, run, jump—but he or she probably stops there. Your doctor doesn't bother telling you *why* you should exercise. Here's a simple explanation. Let's take a runner, for example. You've probably heard of a "runner's high." A runner runs for several miles and, at the end of his exercise, he ends up with a euphoric feeling, a feeling of calm, peacefulness, and well-being. That's because exercise releases hormones called endorphins in the brain.

When you're depressed, there's a depletion of endorphins. Doctors can prescribe medication that will chemically change the brain's hormonal balance so that you won't feel depressed anymore. But a "runner's high" does exactly the same thing: It elevates the level of these hormones . . . only it does it naturally. Again, it's not the running that raises the endorphin level; it's the running that produces the deep breathing and higher oxygen levels that raises the level of hormones. So if you can solve the problem without medication, my advice is do it.

Deep breathing has also been shown to benefit one of the most common, recurring ailments known to mankind: headaches. These are very often caused by a restriction in the muscle tissue, which not only limits the blood supply but also holds the nerves in a tense position and eventually causes a headache. The next time you feel a headache coming on, before reaching for a pain reliever, try taking ten deep, diaphragmatic breaths. See what a difference it makes.

Oxygen and Smoking

Think about people you know who smoke and you'll be able to answer this question right away. Do they look older than they are? The answer is probably yes and I'm going to tell you why. When you smoke, you rob your body of 50 percent of the oxygen it's supposed to have. That's because the chemicals in cigarettes eat up the oxygen in the system. With only half the oxygen you're supposed to have in your body, your cells begin to starve. They can't grow the same way. You lose the suppleness, elasticity, and color in your skin because one-third of the body's blood supply circulates through the skin at all times. The skin is the body's largest organ and with only half the oxygen supply getting to the skin, because blood is the transportation system for oxygen, you're in trouble. And you can't help but look bad, not to mention what those chemicals are doing to your lungs and the rest of your organs.

Paul Bragg says the following about smoking in his book *Super Power Breathing For Super Energy.* "Smoking introduces two deadly poisons into the body, arsenic and carbon monoxide. Nicotine is also poison and immediately affects lung function and constricts your cardiovascular system. It destroys Vitamin C, which is vital to your health and immune system. In twelve hours of not smoking, nicotine blood levels fall and heart and lungs begin healing."

According to Bragg, of the 50 million smoking Americans, one-third to one-half will die from smoke-related diseases. Smoking creates a desire for caffeine and sugar and twice as many smokers drink alcohol than non-smokers. Clinical evidence proves that smokers have a far greater incidence of cancer of the lungs, larynx, pharynx, esophagus, mouth, colon, rectum, and breast.

And here's another double whammy. Your cells are starved of oxygen because you are smoking on top of your normal shallow breathing. You feel tired and draggy. So you start smoking more because you feel you're missing something and you think another cigarette is going to satisfy that need, which is the oxygen depletion in our bodies. But that cigarette just exacerbates the problem you already have, and you've just shot yourself in the foot.

When you do a system like BodyFlex, you'll be helping your lungs go back to what they used to be. You can help clean them out and straighten them up and get them looking good again. And you can get the elasticity, color, and suppleness back to your skin. Right off the bat, from day one, you'll have more oxygen in your system, which of course decreases the desire to smoke because you're satisfying the need for oxygen in a natural way. The more oxygen you have in your system, the less you're going to feel that urge to put more oxygen into the system, so slowly but surely, your desire to smoke will diminish altogether. It's no coincidence that one of the largest and most successful stop-smoking clinics in the world—the Schick Centers—teach deep breathing as the only solution.

Common sense should tell you that you can't undo all the horrific damage of smoking even with BodyFlex, but I hope you'll use BodyFlex as part of your overall wellness program. Use it to get yourself smoke-free for life so you can really be healthy.

Oxygen and Arthritis

Detoxification is also an important process involved in physical ailments such as arthritis. Medical research on arthritis indicates that oxygen can help normalize the joints affected by arthritis and rheumatism. As a matter of fact, if you have arthritis, you probably can attest to the fact that when it rains, your joints hurt more. That's because moisture has replaced some of the oxygen in the air. Lack of oxygen to the joints and toxins in the joints can cause pain. We know that detoxification of the body occurs when you introduce oxygen into the system. You can use BodyFlex to help get rid of toxins and improve the poor circulation that prevents enough oxygen from reaching the joints.

The beauty of deep aerobic breathing exercises, such as BodyFlex, is that they can be done in a stationary position, either sitting or standing, so many people with arthritis pain can participate with their doctor's blessing. This exercise program increases oxygen in the body, thereby increasing circulation to the joints, which activates the lymph system to get rid of the toxins while also elevating the body's own natural painkillers, the endorphins.

Oxygen and Cancer

Cancer is a matter of grave concern in our country. Yet it may surprise you to know that we've known for over sixty years what causes it. Dr. Otto Warburg, the German physiologist, won the Nobel Prize in medicine twice, the first time in 1931 for discovering the cause of cancer. Dr. Warburg stated, "Cancer has only one prime cause. The prime cause of cancer is the replacement of normal oxygen respiration of body cells by anaerobic (lacking in oxygen) cell respiration." In other words, the growth of some cancer cells is initiated by a relative lack of oxygen. They cannot live in an oxygen-rich environment.

Cancer can be viral, bacterial, or environmental. It can be initiated by a lack of oxygen to the cells, lack of nutrition, chemicals, X rays, etcetera. Scientists believe that we all have cancer cells in our bodies. They don't all become full-blown cancer because the white cells of our immune system get rid of them. It makes sense to me that doing whatever we can to keep our immune system strong, including aerobic activity like BodyFlex, can help ward off cancer.

Oxygen and Respiratory Therapy

A couple of years ago, I held a big seminar at one of the hotels in Las Vegas. I had a radio show for two years in the city and I would invite the general public to come and hear me speak about the BodyFlex program. This particular night, I had a group of about eight men who sat right in the front row. And as I was giving my talk and asking the audience for questions, one of these gentlemen stood up and just started in with one question after another. Well, I came to find out that this man had been director of respiratory therapy for Life Therapy, the largest respiratory therapy clinic in the state of Nevada. Gerard Marshall had been the leader for the past eighteen years. He and the other seven doctors stayed and learned the BodyFlex system. They were so impressed with it that they said it was the best system they had ever seen in the field of spirometry, a fancy medical word for breathing. Gerard now gives out copies of my videotapes to his patients.

"I've been a registered respiratory therapist for seventeen years, and I feel that I'm pretty much an expert on breathing," says Marshall in an interview with my cowriter. Marshall was formerly an associate with County LAC-USC Women's Hospital in Los Angeles and with Whittier Presbyterian Hospital in Whittier, California. "I believe strongly in incentive spirometry, which is coordinated deep breathing to hyperinflate the lungs to combat atelectasis [collapsing of the lungs]. The lungs are made up of millions of air sacs called alveoli and when they are inflated properly, they freely exchange oxygen (in) and carbon dioxide (out). But any injury or illness that puts you in bed is going to deflate your lungs. Therefore, you will have less oxygen to power the body. It's like a car running out of gas.

"When I came upon Greer's program, I found a way to coordinate incentive spirometry with rehabilitative medicine. The BodyFlex breathing technique, the abdominal lift, and the exhalation procedure is an activity people can do while they are bedridden. It is the first step to getting them out of bed because BodyFlex develops the trunk muscles, which is the beginning of whole body recovery. And you can't tell people to walk when their lungs aren't inflated. BodyFlex is an excellent tool for clinical respiratory therapists and for rehabilitation medicine therapists as well."

Marshall, by the way, has also tried BodyFlex himself for weight and inch loss. After doing the program faithfully every day for one month, he reports that he lost thirty pounds and "tons" of inches. He says he has even flattened his once large and protruding stomach.

"If people in this country would do this program, they would have no problem with fat at all and they could eat what they want," he says. "We carry more weight from our neck to our groin than anywhere else in the body and we also have more muscle mass there than anywhere else. Greer's program creates an oxygen surplus so that those muscles are given all the oxygen they need so that they can be toned."

O*xygen and Wound Healing*

"There's a lot in the literature about oxygenation in terms of wound healing and in mental well-being and energy levels as well," says Barry Markman, M.D., Las Vegas–based plastic surgeon, award-winning researcher on fat management, and medical adviser to BodyFlex. In an interview with me and my cowriter, Dr. Markman explained, "The concept of super-oxygenation has been around for a long time in hyperbaric oxygenation. Hyperbaric chambers are oxygen-pressurized tanks that drive the oxygen through the skin and into the muscle, healing wounds fifteen times faster than when they are left to the body's own devices, wounds that even surgery can't help. Athletes use it all the time. That's why you see a football player with a serious injury back out on the field in three weeks. This super- or hyper-oxygenation is applicable in Greer's regimen. I can attest to the efficacy of the program because I do it myself and I think it's excellent. It could be a new horizon in terms of an individual type of hyperbaric exercise because it's been shown to work very well in terms of healing and relaxing the body."

Oxygen and HIV/AIDS

They do oxygen therapy in the United States with people who have AIDS and HIV because HIV is a virus. In fact, there's a very famous athlete in our country who, as part of his state-of-the-art treatment, went through almost two years of oxygen therapy, where they took large amounts of blood from the person, saturated it with oxygen, and then transfused it back into him. They have found for the first time ever that the HIV virus is undetectable in this man. I think it's very telling that someone with access to the finest medical treatment available had oxygen therapy as part of his treatment.

How Oxygen Rids the Body of Toxins

You've been hearing me talk a lot about how oxygen rids the body of toxins. Now I want to explain how that happens. First, our bodies eliminate toxins through the lymph system.

What exactly is the lymph system? Here is Alec Borsenko's description of what this system does:

"The lymphatic system—and you have four times more lymph than blood—carries waste from the body so that it can be eliminated. You have millions of lymph nodes all over your body, with the main groups being in the groin, back of the knee, and the armpit areas. They are like holding tanks for waste, which is gotten rid of by your white cells, your immune system. To give you a better idea of what this lymphatic system is all about, I make the following analogy: What would happen to your house if the garbage man didn't come for four months? You'd have infestation and bugs. That's what happens to the body if the lymph doesn't move. The lymph system is the most important system in the body because if it's not working properly, you are going to be sick all the time. And if it's ever shut down, you're going to be dead within twenty-four hours. The lymph system is the dump truck of the body. The toxins circulate through your system and then they have to land somewhere. Guess where they land? They land in the lymph nodes, and if the lymph isn't moving, the nodes become sore and swollen. There has to be some way to get those toxins out of the body. Very deep breathing will move the waste from lymph node to lymph node so that the white blood cells can get rid of the toxins. And what happens if we don't find a way to release them? The dump truck, or lymph nodes, will overflow and start recirculating these toxins back into the system, back into the bloodstream. That's why people are constantly sick. It's because the lymph system is all jammed up.

"BodyFlex moves your lymph system dramatically so that it purifies all waste," says Borsenko. "It's because you are deep breathing during this exercise, and deep breathing, we know now, is what drives the lymphatic system."

In 1979 Dr. C. Samuel West, D.N., N.D., P.M.D., world-renowned lymphologist, and chemist, attended the Eighth International Congress of Lymphology in Montreal, Canada. Dr. West said, "Through deep breathing, you can activate the lymphatic vessels to help pull out all the dead cells, poisons, and excess water." Dr. West advises his patients to breathe deeply to speed the body's healing. (For more information on his books, call 1-800-975-0123.)

Up until 1981, all the experts thought that exercise—moving the muscles—was what triggered the lymph system to get rid of toxins in the body. That year, a group of thirteen doctors from around the world were brought to Italy to conduct an experiment called the Dry State Study. This team of doctors was led by the guru of physiology, Dr. Arthur Guyton, who writes physiology textbooks for medical students. He wanted to determine at what stage in the exercise process the lymph system became activated.

The lymph system is centered in the thoracic area (that's the middle of the chest for those of us who skipped medical school) and when it activates, the lymph comes up through a hoselike structure that connects all the nodes. (The majority of the millions of nodes are in the upper body; your armpit is the king of the lymph nodes.) The doc-

tors hooked an athlete up to monitor him and they pho-
tographed the lymph system for the first time ever. They
told him to walk on a treadmill and they had him walking
and walking and walking . . . and the lymph system stayed
still. So they told him that he had to do more strenuous exercise to kick the lymph system into gear. They had him
doing everything but standing on his head and spitting out
wooden nickels, yet nothing happened.

After about forty-five minutes of strenuous running,
jogging, hopping, and jumping, as well as other exercises,
with nothing happening to the lymph system, the doctors
were perplexed. And the guy was tired, so they told him to
sit down and have a rest and they would start up again in a
little bit. So the athlete sat down and took some deep
breaths from his diaphragm. And guess what happened?
His lymph system just shot up like a geyser, leaving the doctors stunned. They had discovered by accident that it is
deep breathing that triggers the lymph system, not exercise.
It is moving the muscles during exercise that triggers the
deep breathing that triggers the lymph system.

Some of you out there are probably saying to yourself, "Who cares about the lymph system? I just want to
have a skinny waist and a lot of pep." But it all goes together
hand in hand.

Oxygen and Peak Performance

It was in the early eighties that the U.S. Olympic training
committee announced for the first time that they were im-
plementing deep breathing exercises for all Olympic athletes. They said that they had found that these exercises

beefed up the athletes' performance, strength, and stamina to such a degree that they were going to be incorporating deep breathing as part of the regular training process.

If deep breathing does that for an Olympic athlete, what is it going to do for all of us living normal lives? We're not going for the gold, but we all need endurance—we've got kids to take care of, meals to make, laundry to do, errands to run, probably a full-time job on top of all of that. We need endurance just to live a life.

Oxygen and Fat Management

And yes, okay, let's get back to that skinny waist and sag-free butt. "In the area of fat management, this exercise is excellent as well," says Dr. Markman. "Through my studies on fat anatomy, which have been published in the major plastic surgery journals, I have determined that there are actually two different layers of fat, with different metabolic properties, in the stomach and hip and thigh region. That's why it's so hard to lose in these areas and why, up till now, these areas have been considered diet and exercise resistant—no one has been able to unlock the secret of how to get rid of the fat in these areas. Oxygenation in combination with isometric, isotonic, and stretch positions could possibly unlock those layers—the proof is in the pudding. I've lost twenty-five pounds in five weeks as well as major inches in my midsection using BodyFlex. Greer has done it and I think it's revolutionary."

"BodyFlex is a very practical, easy-to-follow, effective program for weight loss and tightening up untoned muscle," says Dr. Carolyn DeMarco, who specializes in women's health and is the author of the Canadian best-seller *Take Charge of Your Body: Women's Health Advisor.* (For more information on this book, call 1-800-387-4761.) "It also increases people's lung capacity; it is very beneficial for people with asthma and other breathing problems. And it only takes fifteen minutes a day so that people can easily put it into their schedules.

"I recommend BodyFlex to my patients who are trying to lose weight, improve their appearance and overall health, or firm up. The combination of stretching and breathing is very effective, with the breathing also being excellent for relaxation as well as increasing oxygen supply to all parts of the body. Most people breathe very shallowly, which can contribute to all kinds of health problems. BodyFlex also strengthens the abdominal muscles and massages the abdominal organs, which helps with bowel problems and constipation."

Dr. Art Davis, former chief of staff and former chairman of the Department of Family Practices for JFK Hospital in California, agrees. In an interview with me and my cowriter, he said, "This program is really impressive. I do it, my wife does it, my kids do it, and my patients do it. And many have lost large amounts of inches and weight. But the common denominator among all of us is three things: First, we function better. If you breathe deeper, you think clearer because you're getting more oxygen to the brain. As the cells get more oxygen, they perform their functions more efficiently. Second, we have a feeling of well-being, we are more energetic, and we look at life in a more positive way. Third, we feel more fit. I do my exercises in a more novel way—I do the breathing while I'm taking a cold shower, which enhances my immune system.

"To me, the breathing and the stretching is a much more holistic approach and the inch and weight loss you get is a very desirable side effect. But how it affects you overall is really very important and can make a tremendous difference in your health and longevity."

Dr. Davis, who while a resident at Loma Linda, a well-known and respected medical school and medical center in California, spent three months in Athens, Greece, working with the Loma Linda heart transplant team, gives an even more detailed explanation of how oxygenation is facilitated through BodyFlex. He explains that by holding your breath for those eight or ten seconds, you build up carbon dioxide in your blood. And when carbon dioxide is built up in the blood, it dilates the arteries, making the cells ready to receive oxygen much more efficiently. In fact, he relates that, in the past, neurologists have administered higher levels of carbon dioxide and oxygen to patients at the same time if they were worried that these patients weren't getting enough oxygen to certain parts of the brain. Again, the carbon dioxide prepared the cells to receive oxygen by dilating the arteries.

So now you have the skinny on BodyFlex and all the things it can do for your overall health. Your body is like an airplane—it can have a perfect engine but if the flaps aren't working, it's going to crash. What good is looking good on the outside if you're not fit on the inside? And, like that plane, all your systems have to be working properly for you to be in optimum health.

Perhaps Dr. Davis sums it up best. "What I would say to the person at home who's overweight, maybe depressed, maybe suffering from a poor self-image, who has little energy, is this: Here's an opportunity for you to make a difference in your life that is inexpensive, that can happen today—you can make a difference *now*. This is a wonderful opportunity. Don't miss it. It's something that can change your life and change it permanently."

Have I got you convinced? Good. Then let's get started.

4.

The
Technique

Breathe Like a Baby

Let me be the first to tell you, it's okay to inhale!

If you are reading this book, I can practically guarantee that you're a shallow, "tidal" breather. You're not drawing in nearly as much air as you could be. If you don't believe me, try this little test. Put one hand on your stomach and another (preferably yours) on your chest. Then take a regular breath. You'll notice that the hand on your chest comes out much farther than the one on your stomach. It should be the other way around.

You were born knowing a better way to breathe. In fact, if you put a baby on the floor and watch him breathe, you will see his stomach going up and down and up and down while his chest stays relatively still. He is belly breathing, or, in other words, doing deep diaphragmatic breathing. The diaphragm is the big bundle of muscle that separates the chest cavity from the rest of the abdomen. It helps keep all the abdominal organs in place and helps the lungs inflate and deflate as we breathe. If you've ever gotten punched in the diaphragm and gotten the wind knocked out of you, you already know how important the diaphragm is for breathing.

As we get older, our bodies become more nervous and our insides, including our diaphragm muscles, start to tighten and tighten and tighten. That's why our breaths typically stop mid-chest and we end up using only 20 percent of our lung capacity, breathing only from the top of our lungs.

To see this even more clearly, lie down on the floor and put a book on your stomach. I would avoid using something like the unabridged dictionary of the modern English language or the complete works of Shakespeare; a paperback will do the trick. Now breathe in through your nose (breathing in through the mouth can create hyperventilation) and exhale through your mouth. Chances are that book will stay put while your chest will rise and fall. After you learn to belly-breathe, when you inhale, you should see the book rise. However, that's going to take some practice; at first your rising chest will be getting in the way of that book, which may stubbornly refuse to move. Keep at it. When you begin to see the book going up and down on your stomach, that means that you have learned to relax your insides and breathe from your diaphragm. You'll be belly-breathing like a baby again.

You Don't Have to Be a Yogi or a Verdi

People have been using deep, diaphragmatic breathing for centuries to improve their health and well-being. A lot of people have asked me if the BodyFlex technique is like yoga. I tell them that in a lot of ways it is actually the opposite of yoga. The only thing that is similar is that there is a focus on deep breathing in both. It's true that yoga is designed to reduce stress in the body, but it utilizes slow, rhythmic breathing that slows down the heart, slows down respiration, and puts you into a deep meditative state. BodyFlex is an aerobic exercise that utilizes a fast inhale and a forceful exhale. It speeds up the heart rate, speeds up your breathing, and puts you into an aerobic state, getting you all geared up.

Opera singers use deep breathing exercises to give them stamina and endurance. I have taught a lot of opera and contemporary singers the BodyFlex technique and they tell me that they can't believe the difference in their lung capacity, the strength in their voices, and their ability to hold notes. Again, the reason people get winded is because they have so little lung capacity. When you work the lungs and the heart and the muscles around them with deep breathing exercises, you increase your lung capacity.

The BodyFlex Technique

Are you ready to learn the BodyFlex accelerated aerobic breathing technique? Before we begin, I want you to stand up, put your hand on your stomach, and take a normal breath. Again, you will feel your chest rise as you inhale; your stomach stays stationary as you breathe in and out. You're about to see a huge difference when you do the BodyFlex method.

Stand with your feet about shoulder width apart. Then pretend you're about to sit down on a chair. Bend forward from the waist, resting your weight on your slightly bent knees with your hands; your rear end is sticking out. Your hands should be about an inch above each knee. Look straight ahead. You'll look a little like an umpire behind home plate waiting for the pitch. This position will make it easier for you to accomplish the final phase of the breathing technique, the "abdominal lift," which I'll explain below.

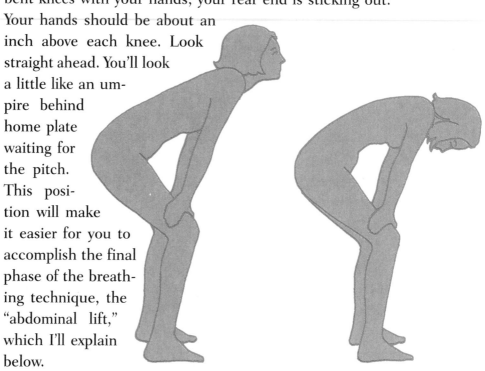

Here are all the steps in the BodyFlex Technique. Then we'll go through each one in greater detail.

The Five Steps of BodyFlex Breathing

1. Blow out all the air in your lungs through your mouth.
2. Inhale quickly through your nose.

3. From your diaphragm, forcefully exhale all the air through your mouth.
4. Holding your breath, do an abdominal lift for a count of 8 to 10.
5. Release the lift and breathe.

Step 1   The first thing you're going to do is exhale all the stale air in your lungs through your mouth. Purse your lips like you're going to whistle and gently and steadily blow the air out until there is nothing left.

Step 2   When your lungs are empty, stop and put your lips together. Keeping your mouth closed, inhale as fast and as sharply as you can through your nose, filling your lungs to capacity. It's almost as though you are sucking in all the air in the room in one breath . . . and it is just as noisy. Imagine you've been underwater too long and you've finally come up for air, you breathe in through your nose as hard and as fast as you can. Imagine pulling that air in as deep as you can; picture it filling your lungs all the way to the bottom. Inhale aggressively; the breathing in is the important part of this exercise because it is the inhalation part of all exercise that accelerates the aerobic process. And, in this case, it is very loud inhalation. If you sound like a Hoover on high, you're probably doing it right.

Step 3   When your lungs are filled to capacity with air and you feel like you can't take in another drop, tip your head up just a little bit. Put your lips together, folding them over your teeth, almost like you're blotting lipstick. You are now going to exhale all the air with a blast from as deep down in the diaphragm as you can. From the "blotting" position, open your mouth wide and dispel the air with as much force as you can. It should sound like you're saying the word *pah*, but it should come from the diaphragm, not from the lips or throat. Getting this deep exhalation right is tricky, and it will probably take you quite a few tries to get the hang of it. The first time you do the exhalation, you might want to cough (from the lungs, not the throat) and keep blowing or belly laughing to initiate the correct technique and to really feel that the sound and the air is coming from deep inside you. You'll know when you're doing the exhalation correctly because you hear a wheezing, whistling sound along with the "pah."

Step 4   Once you have blasted all the air out, close your mouth and hold your breath—and keep holding it through the rest of this step; don't let any of that air sneak back in! Bow your head and then suck your stomach in and up. Picture your stomach and other abdominal organs literally rolling up under your ribs. This is called the "abdominal lift" and it's the part of the technique that will flatten your stomach. (The abdominal lift also massages and stimulates the organs; many people who have had problems with irregularity or bladder control have reported a real fast turnaround.) If you put your hand on your stomach at this point, you will see that it actually feels concave, like the hollow of a bowl right under your ribs. This happens because you have created a vacuum inside you—that's why you were blowing out all that air. Bowing your head down toward your chest simply makes it easier for you to roll your stomach up, since the muscles there are often so weak. Hold your stomach in—still holding your breath—to the count of 8 or 10—counting 1001, 1002, 1003 up to 1008 or 1010. It's during this abdominal lift step that you'll be performing your isotonic or isometric exercises, which I'll explain below.

Step 5   Now let it go; breathe and relax your abdominal muscles. There should be a bit of a gasping sound when you release the breath and feel the air rushing into your lungs. Think of it like a vacuum cleaner. If you put your hand over the hose, when you take it off, you'll hear a kind of gasping, popping, suction sound. What you should hear when you release your breath is a suction sound as the vacuum inside of you is broken. While you were holding your breath in the previous step, you probably felt some pressure—that was air trying to get back into your lungs to fill that vacuum. That's why this is such hard work! Not all my clients, however, make this "popping" sound when they release their breath, but they are still doing the breathing correctly.

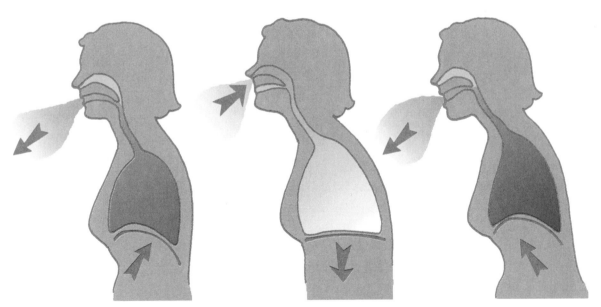

Breathe out through the mouth, in through the nose, then out from the diaphragm.

You Must Remember This

It may take some practice to get the breathing technique down right. You won't be doing it 100 percent correctly the first time you try it, so don't get discouraged. These muscles you use during the abdominal lift may have never had any exercise—they might look a little bit like spaghetti in there. And they've been inside you for, well, however old you are. So you just need a little help. Keep at it, you'll get better at it every day. And here are a few important things to remember:

• Always breathe *in through your nose* and *out through your mouth.*

• If you're not doing the breathing right, you won't be able to get your stomach to roll up. It's kind of like the cog in the wheel—all the parts have to mesh to turn the axle. You need to breathe out hard during Step 1 to make room for all the air you're going to suck in through your nose in Step 2. If you don't exhale forcefully enough in Step 3, you won't be able to create a strong enough vacuum to do a good abdominal lift. So don't phone in any of these steps. Yes, this is breathing, but believe me, if you're doing it right, it's work!

• When you begin doing the "pah" during the exhalation process, you may start coughing. This is to be expected; you're cleaning out your lungs. It will last for maybe a day or two. But with all the secondhand smoke, pollution, and other irritants floating around in the air, your lungs need a lot of clearing out. You may even hear a crackling sound or bring up phlegm and other junk out of your lungs, especially if you're a smoker. But, you know what? In a few days, your lungs are going to start to sound much clearer. And if you're a smoker, deep breathing can help repair the damage caused by the cigarettes. (I hope BodyFlex will also help inspire you to stop smoking if you've got the habit. As I've said, it naturally reduces the desire to smoke.)

• You may feel slightly light-headed when you first start doing the breathing. That's entirely normal—your body has to adjust to the amount of oxygen in your system. If you start feeling downright dizzy, however, stop and sit down. Breathe regularly until the dizziness passes. I don't want anyone keeling over!

• In the beginning, you probably won't be able to hold your breath for very long—that's how you'll know what sad shape your cardiovascular system is in. Some of you may be able to hold your breath for two or three seconds, some for four or five, some for only one. Very few of you will be able to hold your breath for eight to ten seconds on the first go-around. But you'll notice day by day that you will be able to hold your breath longer and longer. After two to three weeks, you should be able to hold your breath easily for fifteen to twenty seconds. When you first start the BodyFlex program, you may also feel winded partway through your fifteen-minute workout. That, too, is perfectly normal. Keep at it to build up your strength and endurance, and pretty soon you'll be able to go through the whole routine without stopping. One of the first things people comment on with this program is that they no longer get winded walking long distances or going up stairs. That's a sure sign that you're doing something good for your cardiovascular system.

• When you begin to learn the positions to go with the breathing, you will find that the breathing is a little more difficult to do lying down. That's because you don't have the force you have when you're standing up, you don't bow your head to your chest, and because you have to make sure you don't lift your head off the floor while doing the abdominal exercises. It's also harder to pull your stomach up under your ribs in this position. In general, the more difficult the position, the more difficult it is to do the breathing. It goes hand in hand. Again, with practice, it'll get a lot easier.

• The best time to do BodyFlex is first thing in the morning upon rising because your stomach has been empty for the longest amount of time. Once we've eaten, all the blood (the transportation system for oxygen, which burns the fat) goes to the digestive system to digest our food. And how can we pull our stomachs up under our rib cages if they're full of food? This exercise is about 40 percent more effective first thing in the morning because the blood supply is going where it's supposed to go and is doing its job with 100 percent effectiveness. It's not busy digesting food.

If you want to do this program after you get home from work, before you have dinner (it's a great energizer for folks who need an instant boost to be there for their kids or to do some other early evening activity), make sure you haven't eaten for at least two hours. But a word of caution: You're always going to have some food in your stomach throughout the day, so BodyFlex is still more effective in the morning.

Assume the Position: Isometric and Isotonic Exercises

I've created isotonic, isometric, and stretch positions to go with the breathing so you can tone your muscles at the same time you're burning the fat. *Isometric* exercises are those that just tighten one group of muscles in opposition to another group of muscles or a stationery object; *isotonic* exercises use the body's own resistance against itself. These forms of exercise have been proven time and time again to be safe and effective.

Straighten your arm out to make a fist. Then squeeze that fist as hard as you can. You should feel your muscles tightening up all the way up the arm. That's an isometric exercise.

Now place your arms in a big round circle in front of your chest, fingers together and elbows up and even with your shoulders and hands. Now push your fingertips against each other. You are going to feel tenseness from your fingertips all the way up your arms—particularly in the bicep area—as well as across your chest. You're using the equal tensions of one hand pressing against the other to create resistance and thereby to create a stress in the inner arm area. That's an isotonic exercise.

The beauty of the entire BodyFlex program is that it is based on simple laws of physics: Oxygen burns fat. Oxygen is carried to various parts of the body through the blood. And when we put a stress or a stretch on a particular part of the body, via isotonic or isometric exercise, more blood travels to that area of stress. Hence, you can burn fat in a specific area and tone muscle simultaneously. If that's not spot reducing, I don't know what is.

Here's how it works: Think about getting hit on the arm, or scraping your leg in a fall. You'll notice that the area turns bright red. Or think about how horribly guilty you feel if you've ever spanked your child and seen your handprint etched in bright red across his or her backside. The telltale mark appears because blood has rushed to that area of stress. In truth, the body cannot decipher whether you're stressing your muscles by hefting a weight in your hand like a bodybuilder, if you've been injured, or if you're doing an isometric exercise. All the body knows is that there is a trauma to a certain part of the body and the message center in the brain records, "Uh-oh, we need blood to that area. We have something going on there; let's shoot some blood over."

I'm not advocating getting spanked to tone your butt! What you have with the BodyFlex program is the ability to direct oxygenated blood to the areas you want to affect by putting a stress or a stretch on that particular area of the body using an isometric, isotonic, or stretch position. When a bodybuilder wants to work on his biceps and build muscle, he uses a weight to create a resistance that puts a stress on the bicep and sends a message to the brain. "Uh-oh, we need blood to the bicep, we need blood to the bicep." As I've said previously, BodyFlex, conversely, doesn't build muscle. Instead of using weights to shorten and bulk up muscle, we use positions that elongate and tone muscle. We lengthen the muscle to become more flexible and agile so we can have bodies that move and bend and stretch as we age.

Let's say you're doing a crunch and are stressing the abdominals. The message center in the brain directs the blood to the abdominals. If you're doing the deep aerobic breathing along with the crunch, then you can burn excess fat in the stomach and ab area while toning the muscles. If you're not doing the breathing, you're doing what 99 percent of the general public does: building bulk instead of flattening and elongating. Their main complaint is that they're doing crunches all the time but their stomachs are getting bigger and harder rather than flatter and trimmer. That's because they're building muscle under fat; without doing aerobic breathing, they can't become aerobic enough to dramatically increase the oxygen to the body to burn fat. So they're just tightening the abdominal muscles under the existing fat layers.

While just the BodyFlex method of breathing, done on a day-to-day basis, will cause your metabolism to accelerate, the exercises in Chapter 6 of this book will enable you to burn fat and tone muscle in those areas where you need it most.

First the Technique, Then the Workout

As with any exercise program, it's a good idea to let your doctor know you're starting BodyFlex.

I recommend that you spend a few days perfecting the BodyFlex technique before you begin the actual workout. You'll want to feel completely comfortable with all five steps—who wants to be flipping pages while they're doing the breathing?—before you add the isometric and isotonic exercises. Out. In. Out. Hold. Relax. To get a sense of your improvement, try the book exercise I described earlier. By the end of a few days with BodyFlex breathing, you should see that book rise higher than your chest. Now that's higher learning!

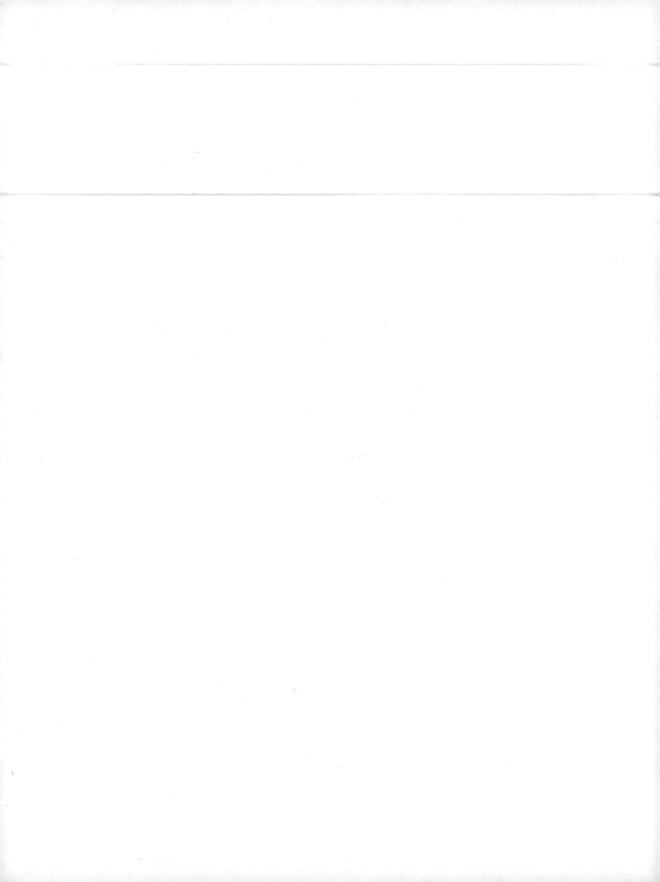

5.

To Breathe or Not to Breathe

That shouldn't even be the question.

In fact, here's a better one: Do you have a treadmill or a bike or a walker or a rider or an ab machine down in the basement or in a corner of your bedroom or in your laundry room collecting dust or being used as a clothes rack for your wet laundry that you don't want to put in the dryer? Or are you one of those people who thinks that becoming lean and fit is going to happen by magic?

Finding the Motivation

When we say that we want to get in shape and we want to do the right thing and we want to look healthier and feel better, we mean it . . . and for the first week or so, we're really on track. We go out and buy ourselves a program of some kind, we join a gym, we do this, we do that. And let me just tell you this: The gyms out there oversell their memberships by about four or five times over capacity because they're counting on you to drop out. And you know what? You do! How many of you reading this book joined a gym at one time? Lots of you. How many are still going? Almost no one.

Why? We lose our motivation. We lose our sense of urgency. We just get into a place of complacency or hopelessness where we think nothing's going to work anyway so why even try. Or, conversely, we become desperate because nothing is working. So, we choose the wrong program, we sign up and spend a fortune, we try crazy diets and everything else, and here we still are—disgusted, discouraged, and still looking, even after all the proposed solutions in the marketplace.

And the bottom line is that whether we're failing because whatever we're trying to do is unrealistic, too expensive, it doesn't work, we don't want to do it, or any or all of the above, we're not doing it and we're in the same boat we've always been in. And with the average dress size in this country being a size 14, that's quite a tanker.

Why I Got Off My Butt

As for me, being an average American woman with three children, I needed and wanted something that was fast, that got me quick results without my having to give up hardly anything, and was cheap. And I wanted something I could do at home because I felt self-conscious. If people thought that my size 16 body was going to be exercising in a G-string down at the local gym, working out with all these muscleheads, they were sadly mistaken. So what I did was nothing at all. I just stayed at home and got fatter and fatter and flabbier and more disgusting and disgusted as the days went by. I continued to buy my clothes from Omar the Tentmaker so that I could camouflage my body and not have to go out and do anything.

Like most other people, I was looking for a magic potion or, at the very least, a fairy godmother who could wave her magic wand and turn me into a thin, trim, beautiful Cinderella-type creature. Every time one of my kids lost a tooth, I considered waiting up for the tooth fairy myself. Then, of course, once I realized that there was no magical way to make my stomach, butt, and thighs disappear, I took my desperate and ill-fated foray into the world of diet, pills, depression, trainers, and exerciserabilia that I told you about earlier. Finally I found the techniques I would later develop into BodyFlex—and, of course, I laughed and made a big joke out of it because, as I said before, I thought that standing still and breathing and losing inches in one week was the dumbest thing I ever heard. Then my life changed. I had been laughing because I didn't understand it. It turned out that I was the dumb one—I just didn't comprehend how it all works.

When I first learned BodyFlex, I wasn't expecting anything—except for it to fail just like always. Nothing else had ever worked, so why should this? I was pushing forty and had failed at every single thing I ever tried to do to help myself. I was flabby as could be. My stomach was so big that I began to think of it as an added appendage, one that moved independently and arrived everywhere I went seconds before I did. I fantasized about just cutting it off.

The only reason I even attempted to learn the BodyFlex technique was that it had worked for someone I knew. And when I lost 10½ inches in my problem midsection the first week on this program, I found myself suddenly loving life. For once in my existence, I had found something that really did work. And I didn't have to give up everything. And I did it without having to go to the gym and have everybody looking at me and saying, "Well, you know what? She's had three kids. What do you expect her to look like?" I didn't want that. I wanted to be by myself like all of you do—you don't like the way you look and the last thing you want to do is flaunt it in front of other people. Especially *fit* people. And who wants to spend all that time driving and parking and changing at the gym—not to mention shelling out for the membership?

The truth is, after I saw the results that first week, I was too scared to *stop* doing BodyFlex, because I thought I'd go right back to being a size 16 with a big fat stomach and people asking me if I was pregnant when I wasn't. Though I didn't want to have to do anything to get myself back into shape, I knew that wishing away the fat and flab wasn't the answer, and I felt that this was the least problematic thing I could do. Even with three young kids, I felt I had fifteen minutes a day to do something good for myself. But I'm going to be honest with you: It was really the fear of getting big again that motivated me into continuing with the program.

We're all afraid, every single one of us. And, with BodyFlex, I don't think a lot of people are afraid that it's *not* going to work, I think they're afraid that it *is* going to work and they'll no longer have excuses for the lacking in their lives, the things an improved appearance and mental attitude can bring. In my seventeen years of doing this program, I've seen some pretty incredible things. I've had people—great big women—come to me and cry and say, "Please will you teach me this? Please, please, please." My classes would be full and I wouldn't have any space left, but I would cram this person into my class because she was so desperate. It never failed—after a week or two, she would call me almost in tears saying, "Oh, I'm so happy, I've lost all these inches. My clothes are starting to hang on me.

Thank God, I've finally found something that's really working for me." Then I'd see this person two months later and she'd have ballooned back up again. And I'd say, "What happened?" And she'd be all sheepish and wouldn't want to talk to me because she had stopped doing BodyFlex.

Aren't You Worth Fifteen Minutes a Day?

I've heard every excuse you could imagine.

- "I'm just too busy."
- "I'm not a morning person."
- "I got a cold and couldn't breathe through my nose, and I just didn't start BodyFlex again when I got well."
- "My husband says I look silly doing BodyFlex."
- "My friend's on this new grapefruit-prunes-chocolate-syrup diet and everyone at the office is trying it."
- "I'm going to start next week, as soon as this big project is over."
- "My girlfriend wants to go on a walking program with me, so we'll do that together instead."
- "The kids won't leave me alone for a second, let alone fifteen minutes."

I listen to this kind of stuff over and over, and you know what I've got to say? *I'm just not buying it.*

My question to everyone is this: When you finally find something that only takes fifteen minutes a day, that has been proven to work, that gives you results the first

week, that is something you can do at home, that is inexpensive, that you don't have to diet with, WHAT'S
WRONG WITH YOU? Aren't you worth fifteen minutes a
day? Why would you stop doing it? If you aren't doing this,
you'd better take a good long look at yourself in the mirror
because I don't know anything that's cheaper, faster, less
painful, more effective, and offers the path of least resistance. And if you're not doing this, you're not going to do
anything, so you better take a good hard look at that 14–16
rear end of yours (try a three-way mirror, that's really scary)
because it's never going to get any smaller unless you get
off it.

So I say this: Take that path of least resistance. Get
on the program. Do what the program says. Measure yourself before you start the program, and after five to seven
days, remeasure. The results will give you the motivation to
keep going—the tape measure doesn't lie. You need five to
seven days, and fifteen minutes a day, that you can invest in
yourself. I don't care what it takes. Roll out of bed, turn on
the coffee, and do your BodyFlex while it's perking. Look,
I'm not a morning person either, but I promise you that if
you can just make yourself start the breathing, within two
or three breaths, you'll feel alert and energized, and you'll
be glad you made the effort. If your husband thinks you
look goofy, remind him of that leisure suit he wore in 1981.
By all means, walk with your girlfriend, but do your
BodyFlex, too. Just say "no" to the latest diet fad—how
many do you need to try before you realize that you already
own all the common sense you need to eat right? Your kids
can be taught to leave you alone when you're in the bathroom; teach them that they've got to let you have your fifteen minutes to exercise. Please don't try to tell me that you
don't have fifteen extra minutes in your day. Think of all the

ways you fritter away that amount of time over the course of a single day. No more excuses! Up to this point, nothing you've tried has worked. It's either this or remain the way you are. And I don't think you want to do that or you wouldn't have picked up this book. You've got to make the commitment to do this for yourself.

BodyFlex Works for Almost Everybody

I've had lots of people tell me, "Look, I wish I could exercise. But I really can't. I've got a medical problem." I understand how hard that can be, but I've got your answer. It doesn't matter if you are fifty years old and have never exercised. It doesn't matter if you are challenged in some way or are in a wheelchair. It doesn't matter if you have a bad back. I've had people with all these problems get results with BodyFlex. We all know that exercise will keep the heart and lungs in peak condition, our bodies strong, and help us to have more energy and live longer. I am a firm believer in getting the maximum results with the least amount of effort. BodyFlex can work for you. It is an exercise program done in a stationary position; it is an accelerated aerobic breathing technique that you can do standing or sitting and it works the heart and lungs and the muscles around them, thereby strengthening them. Combined with the isometric, isotonic, and stretch positions, you will burn body fat and tone muscle simultaneously and also develop flexibility. Of course, as with any exercise program, you should check with your doctor first before doing this.

As I will discuss in the next chapter, this program can be adapted to almost anybody's needs or physical limitations. And, by the way, those of you with back problems may get great relief from doing BodyFlex. A lot of people with bad backs think the problem is that their back muscles aren't strong enough. Wrong! Many back problems result from too-tight, inelastic back muscles and weak abdominal muscles, where the back has to take over the work of the weak abs. This program will strengthen those abdominal muscles and help take the strain off the back.

The bottom line is that BodyFlex will work for practically *everybody.* I've sold more than three million sets of videos (two to a set) to date—all these people can't be wrong. Neither can all the doctors, respiratory therapists, lymphologists, and other medical people who recommend this program to their patients. Neither can all the athletes, authors, models, and entertainers who do BodyFlex. Everyday people, women *and* men, just like you and me, have gotten results. So can you.

Remember: BodyFlex works on pure scientific principle: Oxygen burns fat. Put stress on a particular area of the body, and blood is sent to that area. Blood transports oxygen. And oxygen is vital to our bodies for a whole host of medical reasons as well. It couldn't be any more basic.

$\mathcal{W}$hat Can Slow You Down

There are outside factors, such as medication, that can affect the results of BodyFlex where inch loss is concerned. Thyroid medication, birth control pills, and certain types of antidepressants will *slow down,* not eliminate, the results. These particular medications contain an ingredient that slows the metabolism. And since BodyFlex speeds up the metabolism, you have one fighting against the other. Still, if you do BodyFlex on a consistent basis, the results will come. They just may take a little longer. Remind yourself of this so you won't be disappointed by slower results and use it as an excuse to slack off.

Then there are the people with a naturally slower metabolism, and again, their results will take a little more time. That's why I say most of my clients lose somewhere between 4 and 14 inches that first week in the midsection—stomach, thighs, waist, upper and lower abs—alone. Someone with a very, very slow metabolism might only end up with a 4-inch loss, sometimes less. But, hey, 4 inches in one week is ten times more than you're going to get with any other fitness program that's got you working yourself to death. Of course, results vary, but even at its worst, even with the slowest metabolism in the world, you're still going to get results eventually.

For all you normal, average people out there—which is the majority of us—here's some interesting information. There was a two-week study done in August 1997 by Trotta and Associates in Orange County, California, to offer market research on this program. The results on a group of women and men between ages thirty and fifty using Body-Flex showed that most had lost on average more than 8 inches in all from their waist, hips, thighs and arms by the end of the second week. Some had lost between 16 and 17½ inches! And you know what? Every one of them, without exception, before they started it, thought there was no way the program would work. But some had tried so many things that hadn't worked that they thought it sounded sensible enough and was unusual enough to try. I've read hundreds and hundreds of letters from people who have tried BodyFlex and loved the results. Results don't lie.

For many of us, woman or man, our metabolism starts to slow down when we reach thirty-five or forty.

That's why we put on weight even though we're eating the same way we always have and are doing the same old things. So what we do is diet. But did you know that dieting by itself slows the metabolism? If you're used to having 2,500 calories a day and you go down to 1,500, your body begins trying to save every calorie and it slows the metabolic rate down because it is starving itself. You deprive your body and it deprives you right back.

So you have to exercise to increase your metabolism. What we need to do instead of eating less—because we've all been held hostage by food for such a long time, our whole society revolves around food—is to forget about food and learn to look at our fitness level and our weight level in terms of metabolism. If you speed up your metabolism, you will burn calories faster and get rid of that excess poundage. The answer is not to eat less and starve yourself; it's to change your metabolism. Professional weight loss counselors will tell you it's all about metabolism. And remember, the only way to change your metabolism is through aerobic breathing.

But please don't get all caught up with weight loss. That's not what BodyFlex is all about. It's about toning and shaping and feeling more energetic, more vibrant. Who cares what you weigh if you feel draggy? I'd like you to see your results in terms of a higher energy level and fewer belt notches. Scales aren't part of my plan, and they shouldn't be part of yours.

$\mathcal{M}$ake the Right Choice

Now that you understand how it all works, you can make a much more intelligent decision. And that intelligent decision should be BodyFlex, the path of least resistance. Basically we all want the same thing, it's just a matter of how we're going to get it. Very few women want to look like a mud wrestler. Very few women want to look like a female Charles Atlas. Most of us don't want 23-inch biceps and 35-inch quads. We don't want something unrealistic. We just want to look better and feel better.

We also want to be limber, flexible, and have a wider range of motion. Doctors will always tell you, "Keep limber." Think about poor Aunt Mary. She breaks a hip, she goes into the hospital and either she doesn't come out or she heads for the nursing home for a nice, long—maybe even permanent—stay. She doesn't get out because she doesn't heal up right. The reason she got hurt is brittle bones. And the reason she fell in the first place? No range of motion or flexibility, because she hasn't done any exercise. We want to be able to bend and move and stretch. And BodyFlex will get us there. This is probably one of the most important things when it comes to aging, because falling is one of the most common things to happen to people as they get older. Let's do what we can so that that doesn't happen to us. We don't want to miss a step like poor Aunt Mary. We need to take every step we possibly can to stay looking good, youthful, flexible, and agile for as long as we can.

To breathe or not to breathe? Now you know the answer: BodyFlex.

6

The BodyFlex Workout

efore we begin, here's a word of advice: DO try this at home.

BodyFlex is designed for the average person who doesn't have much time, who doesn't have the desire to go to the gym for two or three hours to exercise, who may have physical limitations or be challenged in some way, and who wants results fast. Let's face it, we've moved from the Pepsi generation into the Now generation. If we don't see results *now*, forget it.

Get Ready

So what is it you need to get with the program? Just fifteen minutes a day, first thing in the morning. Remember, you want to do BodyFlex on an empty stomach. However, you can have a glass of water or a cup of coffee since they're liquid and don't have to be digested. But it's best if you can just hop out of bed and get started. What should you wear? Your pj's will suffice. So will any other form of attire (or nonattire) you are comfortable in, as long as it's not binding and you can stretch and bend in it. If you feel more juiced up wearing workout clothes, that's fine, but you don't need any special clothes or special equipment. You don't have to leave your house, your cat, your refrigerator . . . or better yet, if you prefer to work out with the BodyFlex videotapes, your TV set.

Okay, I lied. You do need one piece of special equipment: You *will* need a tape measure. It is most critical to be able to see with your own eyes, on a weekly basis, how many inches you're losing. That's why, before you learn to do this program, you need to measure five very specific areas in your midsection: the waist, upper abs (2 inches above the waist), lower abs (1 inch below the belly button), the hips (around the bikini line), and the thighs (around the widest part). A word of caution: If at all possible, *don't* measure yourself. Try to have someone else measure you to get the most accurate reading. You can't measure yourself properly when you're bending over to look at your midsection areas—bending over adds inches. However, if you don't have a friend or significant other to help out, or if you'd really rather

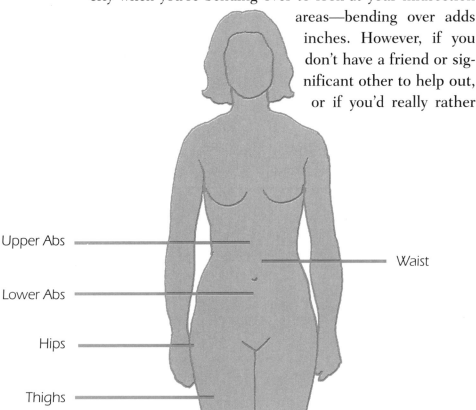

Upper Abs

Waist

Lower Abs

Hips

Thighs

keep your dimensions under wraps, then just do it yourself. It's better to measure yourself than to skip the measurements and use it as an excuse not to do BodyFlex.

What's motivating about BodyFlex is that, in one to seven days, if you're doing the program correctly, you will see dramatic inch loss—many of my clients lose 4 to 14 inches the first week—in this midsection area, which is the biggest problem area for both women and men. Keep a log of your measurements for one month, week by week. Also, don't measure yourself more than once a week. (If you get bloating before your period, note this on your measurement log, because it'll affect the results. You won't be able to see the true inch loss until after the bloating goes away.) Take a baseline measurement before you start the program, then measure seven days later, then seven days after that, and so on. You'll see the quick results with your own two eyes. Now that's instant gratification!

	Starting Measurement	1st Week	2nd Week	3rd Week	4th Week
Upper Abs					
Waist					
Lower Abs					
Hips					
Thighs					

Another good thing to do before you begin BodyFlex is to take a pair of pants that you know are too tight and uncomfortable, or that you can't get over your balloon hips or pouchy stomach, and set them aside. At the end of each

week, try that same pair of pants on. You'll find that each
week you'll be able to get them up a little higher, close them
a little more, and that they are becoming looser and looser.
The tape measure doesn't lie and neither do your clothes.
It's also another great motivator.

As I've stated before, anyone on my team doesn't
worry about the scale. I told you that I weigh 151 pounds
and although I am 5 feet 10 inches tall, I know people my
height who weigh 150 pounds and wear a size 14. Again,
this program is about losing body fat and inches simultaneously, and inch loss is where it's at.

The important thing to remember is that you do the
five-step breathing technique you learned in Chapter 4—
blow out, inhale, blast out the air, hold your breath, tuck
your head (except when lying down), suck your stomach
in—and then once you do the abdominal lift, you immediately go into the exercise position, holding that position—and your breath—to the count of 8 or 10.
And hereafter, when I refer to "doing the
breathing," I am referring to the entire
five-step process before going into
the exercise position.

The BodyFlex Workout

Are you ready for the BodyFlex workout? I'll explain each position in detail. When you first begin the workout, you'll need to refer to the specific pages for each exercise. When you become more proficient, you can simply turn to p. 123 for my "cheat sheet" picture summary of the workout; this quick reference will save you some page flipping.

1. THE LION

*T*he unique thing about BodyFlex is that it is the only exercise program I have ever seen that works not only the body but also the face and neck. And I think that's critical because who cares if your body looks twenty-five if your face looks seventy with a double chin and saggy jowls? You want to have a toned face and neck right along with your body. One third of the body's blood supply circulates through the skin at all times—the skin is the largest organ. When you increase oxygen to the blood, when it circulates through the skin, you're delivering nutrients to the skin. Oxygen gives the skin more elasticity, vibrancy, suppleness, and tone.

Starting position: Begin in the usual standing position, feet 12 to 14 inches apart, hands resting an inch above the knees, looking as though you're about to sit down. Do your breathing, hold your breath, suck your stomach up, and go into the exercise position.

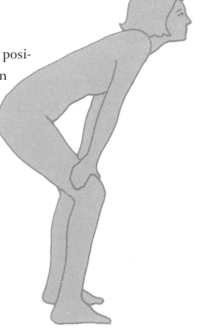

Exercise position: This position is for the face, cheeks, under the eyes, and the creases around the mouth and nose. It comes from a yoga position, but it's done a little bit differently. In yoga, you open your mouth and lips wide and it's just a big old lion's mouth. This is not what we want, because what that does is create more and deeper creases in the face. In our Lion, you first make a small O.

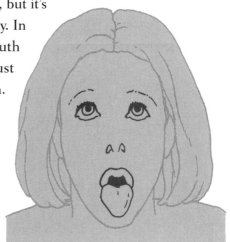

Then, you open your eyes real wide and look up (which works the muscles under the eyes); as you do this, you pull the O down (creating a stretch in the cheek area and in the crease area along the nose), making it a low O and sticking your tongue all the way out (this works the area under the chin and down the neck), still keeping the O small. Hold this position for the count of 8. Do this five times.

DO'S AND DON'TS

- Don't open your mouth real wide. The O should be small, like you're surprised.

- When you stick your tongue out of the small, low O as far as it will go, you should feel a pull from under your eyes all the way down to your chin.

- For this exercise, you can either stay in the basic breathing stance the entire time or you can stand up after your stomach rolls up. Do the facial position while holding your breath to the count of 8, and come back to the basic breathing stance as soon as you release your breath.

2. THE UGLY FACE

The neck is the tattletale area of the body—it reveals your age. You might also be battling a wrinkled "turkey" neck. Plus, every person past the age of thirty-five is starting to worry about a double chin. And anytime you're carrying around a little bit of excess body fat, you're going to have a double chin. The first area on a person's body that will respond to exercise is beneath the chin. There's usually not a lot of fat under there; it's usually just gravity and sagging skin. So if we want to get beautiful, first we're going to have to get real ugly.

Starting position: You might want to try the Ugly Face alone before you put it together with the breathing. Start by standing straight; put your bottom teeth over your top teeth (in what a dentist would call a severe underbite) and then pucker up to kiss somebody (you might want to stay away from any amorous monkeys since you will resemble one yourself). As you pucker up, you're going to jut your neck way out like a stubborn bulldog until you feel a stretch on your neck. Then you're going to tilt your head up and pretend you're going to kiss the ceiling. You should feel a stretch from the tip of your chin all the way down to your breastbone. Don't be surprised the next morning if you feel as if someone slugged you in the neck, because these are muscles that never get worked. Once you've mastered the Ugly Face (and understand how it lives up to its name), you can put it together with the rest of the exercise. For your starting position, assume the basic standing stance, with legs apart, hands above the knees, and your butt out like you're about to sit down. Do your breathing, hold your breath, suck your stomach up, and go into the exercise position.

Exercise position: Assume the neck and chin position described above, stand up straight, with your arms pushing straight back behind you like you're on a diving board (this is for balance) while you reach your chin up to the ceiling. Your feet should be flat on the ground. Do this five times, holding your breath to the count of 8 each time.

DO'S AND DON'TS

- Don't close your mouth—put your bottom teeth over your top teeth, then pucker like you're making monkey lips.

- Don't stand on your toes when you reach for the ceiling. Not only could you lose your balance, you won't get as much of a stretch.

- Make sure you return to the basic breathing stance before doing the next repetition. Catch your breath and repeat.

3. THE $\mathcal{S}$IDE STRETCH

$\mathcal{S}$ay good-bye to waist and side flab with this exercise.

Starting position: Stand in your basic breathing position—legs shoulder width apart, knees bent with hands about an inch above each knee, rear end sticking out like you're about to sit down on a chair, head looking forward. Do the breathing, hold your breath, suck your stomach up, then go into the exercise position.

Exercise position: Drop your left arm so that your elbow rests on your bent left knee. Take your right leg and slide it out and stretch it to the side, toes pointed and foot resting on the carpet. Your weight should be on the bent left knee. Now raise your right arm and stretch it over your head, coming right up over your ear, stretching and stretching so that you feel a pull along your side from your waist up to the under-arm area. Keep your arm straight and close to your head. Hold to the count of 8, then release your breath. Do three times on the left side, then reverse and repeat three times on the right side.

DO'S AND DON'TS

- Don't bend the elbow of the arm you're reaching over the top of your head or you won't get the necessary stretch. Just reach and stretch.

- Make sure the toes of the outstretched leg are pointed so that you give yourself a real good stretch.

- Keep your body in good alignment. Try not to lean forward out of the stretch.

- If you're in the right position, you'll look slightly like a Roman discus thrower.

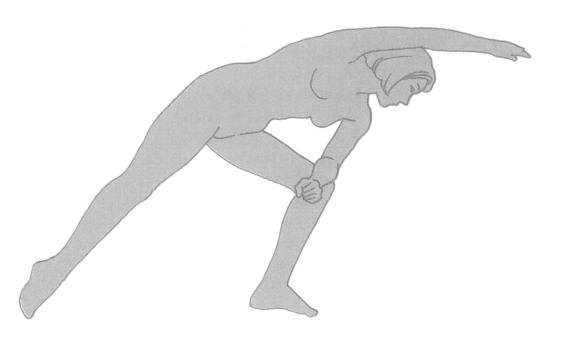

4. THE BACK $\mathcal{L}$ EG EXTENSION

*I love this position because it works one of the parts of me
that needs the most help. My butt was so flat and saggy
that I didn't know if I could ever get it into shape. But this
bun shaper did the trick.*

Starting position: Get down on your hands and knees. Now drop to
your elbows. Stretch one leg out straight behind you, knee straight,
foot flexed with toes pointing down and resting on the floor. Your
weight should be on your elbows and arms, which are straight in front
of you, palms down. Your head is up and you're looking straight ahead.
Do your five-step breathing all the way through: exhale, inhale, blast
it out, hold your breath, tuck your head down, and suck your stomach
in. Once you've rolled up your stomach, hold it and go right into position.

Exercise position: Take the leg that's straight back and raise it as high
as you can, foot still flexed down. Pretend you have your life savings in
between your butt cheeks and squeeze your rear end to put a stress on
the gluteus maximus area. Hold that position and your breath and
squeeze, squeeze, squeeze to the count of 8. Release your breath and
bring your leg down. Do three repetitions with this leg and then three
with the other leg.

DO'S AND DON'TS

- Don't point your toes during this exercise. If you do, you change the flow of the blood (which is carrying the fat-burning oxygen) and direct it into the calf area. And we don't want to work the calf right now; we want to work the glut (affectionate term for the big muscle in the butt). Keep your foot flexed down at all times.

- Keep the leg totally straight. Don't let your knee bend at all, again to put the stress on the glut.

- Never, ever do this exercise unless you are on your elbows. Don't do it on your hands and knees or you'll end up hurting your back.

- For this, as with all the following exercises, don't waste valuable time getting into position once you have sucked in your stomach, since you won't begin your count of 8 until you are in the actual exercise position. Move swiftly from the abdominal lift to the exercise position.

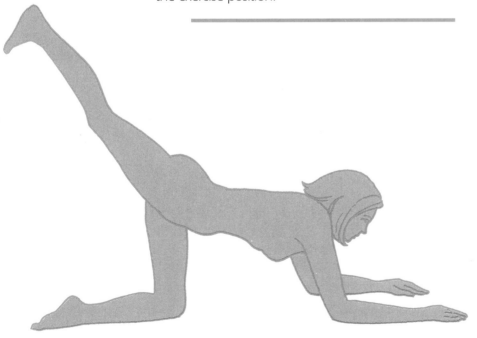

5. THE SEIKO

I named this next exercise the Seiko because in Japanese the word seiko means flame. And this exercise feels like a flame on your upper thighs when you do it. It is designed for the hip area.

Starting position: Get on your hands and knees and position your right leg straight out to the side at a right angle to your body, your right foot resting on the floor. Do your breathing, hold your breath, suck your stomach up, and go into the exercise position.

Exercise position: Raise the extended leg up to hip level, like a dog "watering" a fire hydrant, and pull it forward toward your head. Keep your leg straight. For this exercise, your toes can be pointed or straight; it really doesn't matter. Just hold it there for a count of 8. Release your breath and lower your leg back to the extended position on the floor. Do this exercise three times on each side.

DO'S AND DON'TS

- Don't bend the knee of the lifted leg—that takes the focus off the inner thigh.

- Try to get your leg up as high as you can. Most people will only be able to lift it off the ground about 4 inches on the first go-round.

- Keep your arms straight during the lift. It's okay to tilt your body a little to the side opposite of the lift to help you keep your balance, but try to keep your body as straight as possible.

---

6. THE $\mathcal{D}$IAMOND

This exercise will help get rid of that jiggling flab on the inside of your arms and give your biceps a lovely rounded look.

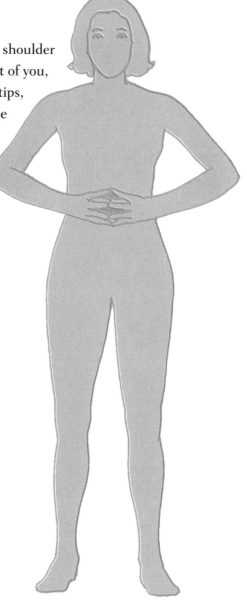

Starting position: Stand with your feet about shoulder width apart and hold your arms in a circle in front of you, keeping your elbows up and putting your fingertips, fingers spread, together. Round your back a little so that you can keep your elbows up and have only your fingertips—not your palms—touching each other. Do your breathing, hold your breath, suck your stomach up, and go into the exercise position.

Exercise position: Now push your fingertips together as hard as you can. You will feel the muscle tension go from both wrists all the way up to the arms and around the chest. Maintain the pressure on your fingertips for a count of 8. Then release your breath. Do three repetitions.

DO'S AND DON'TS

- Make sure just your fingertips are touching.
- Don't drop your elbows. If you drop them, you put the pressure solely on your chest instead of your upper arms.

7. THE ROWBOAT

This next exercise is for the inner thighs, so that when we stop walking, our inner thighs can stop with us. This is a great way to tighten up all that flab on the inner thigh area.

Starting position: Sit on the ground with your legs extended as far apart as you can get them in a very wide and open V. With heels on the ground, flex your toes up, and rock them outward so you get an additional stretch on the inner thigh. Put your hands behind you on the floor, supporting yourself with straight arms. Do the five-step breathing. Once you tuck your head and suck your stomach up, hold your breath and go into position.

Exercise position: Take your hands from behind your back and, bending from the waist, place your hands on the floor in front of you. Keeping your fingers on the carpet, "walk" them farther and farther out, leaning forward more and more as you go. You will feel a stretch on the inside of your thigh. Hold for a count of 8. Breathe out, put your hands in back of you and start again. Repeat this exercise three times.

DO'S AND DON'TS

- This should be a gentle stretch. As you are leaning farther and farther out, walking your fingers, don't bounce—that can cause injury. Simply stretch. Reach and stay there, then lean a little bit more and stay there, lean a little more and stay there, elongating and stretching those inner thigh muscles. Relax into the stretch; don't force it.

- You can also do this exercise using a table leg. Straddle a table leg, again with your legs in as wide a V as possible. As part of your starting position, grab the table leg (which should be about a foot from your chest) with both hands and after you've done your breathing and then held your breath, pull your chest forward using the table leg and then hold for a count of 8.

- If you don't feel a stretch in the inner thigh, it means your legs are not in a wide enough V. If you haven't stretched in a while, it may take some effort to widen your V. Keep with it.

- Try not to bend your knees. Bending takes the focus off the stretch.

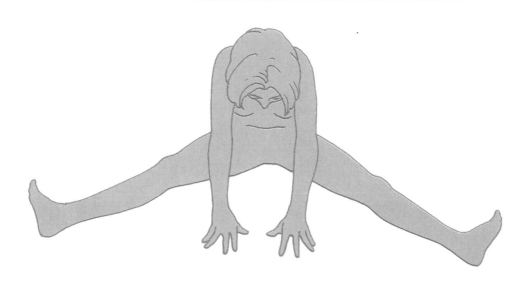

8. THE $\mathcal{P}$RETZEL

*ere's one to tone the outer thighs. It will also help the
waist area and is terrific if your lower back feels tight.*

Starting position: Sit on the floor with your legs
crossed at the knees, left knee on top of the right.
Keep your lower legs as horizontal and as straight as
possible. Place your left hand behind your back
and grab your left knee, which is on top, with
your right hand. Do your breathing, hold your
breath, suck your stomach up, and go into the
exercise position.

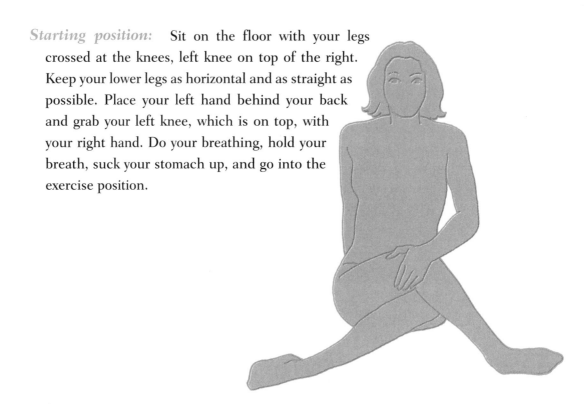

Exercise position: With your weight resting on your left hand, use your right hand to pull the left knee up and toward you as far as you can while twisting your body, at the waist, to the left until you are looking behind you. You should feel a stretch in the outer thigh as well as in the waist. Hold for a count of 8 to 10. Release your breath and start again. Do this exercise three times with the left leg on top, then do it three times on the other side, crossing your knees so that the right knee is on top, placing your right hand behind your body, then pulling your knee up and forward as far as you can with your left hand as you twist your body, at the waist, to the right until you are looking behind you.

DO'S AND DON'TS

- When pulling your knee up and forward, pull it as close to your chest as you can.
- When you're twisting at the waist, try to see as far behind you as you can. You'll really feel the difference in the stretch.

9. THE HAMSTRING $\mathcal{S}$ TRETCH

his exercise is for the area at the back of the thigh, which is one of women's biggest problem areas, because that's where they start to develop cellulite, those little deposits of fat that re- semble cottage cheese or orange peels (which could conceivably lessen your desire to do lunch).

Men are also very inflexible in this area—called the hamstrings, the powerful muscles that run down the back of the legs— be- cause most of them have worked out so much that their ham- strings are short and tight. Try this experiment right now. Stand up straight, then bend over from the waist while keeping your legs straight and try to touch your toes. Chances are your fingertips ended somewhere around your calves. This is a sign of a tight hamstring. This exercise will stretch out the hamstrings while toning up the muscle and therefore the skin. Here's an occasion to really ham it up.

Starting position: Lie flat on your back. Put your legs straight up in the air. Flex your feet so that they are flat. (You can put a pillow under your bottom if you have a bad back.) Reach up and grab the back of each upper calf with your hands, keeping your elbows up. (If you can't reach your upper calves, behind the knees will do.) Keeping your head and back on the floor, do your breathing exer- cises—exhale, inhale, blast out, hold your breath, suck your stomach up (remember, when you are lying down you don't tuck your head before doing your abdominal lift). As soon as you suck your stomach up, go into position.

DO'S AND DON'TS

- Try not to bend your knees, though in the beginning you may have to because you are not as flexible as you may have thought. Make a long, lean line from butt to foot your goal. Each day you'll get better and better at it.

- Don't rock your rear end off the floor, because that defeats the purpose of the exercise. The stretch has to come in your hamstring, and if your bottom lifts up, the stretch won't be concentrated where you need it.

- Keep your head on the ground at all times; don't let it lift off the ground while you're holding your count.

- Keep you feet flattened on the bottom.

Exercise position: While keeping your legs straight, use your hands to gently move your legs toward your head, as you pull them closer and closer, try to keep your rear end on the floor so that the stress is on your hamstring. You'll feel a stretch back there that you may never have felt before because you have probably never worked that area before. Hold the position to the count of 8. Release your breath and bring your legs back to the straight up position, feet flexed, hands around the calves. Do this exercise three times.

10. THE ABDOMINAL $\mathcal{C}$ RUNCH

$\mathcal{H}$*ere's one for the upper and lower abs.*

Starting position: Lay on your back, flat on the floor, legs straight. Now pull your legs up so that your knees are bent and your feet are flat on the floor, 12 to 14 inches apart. Reach your hands straight up in the air as if you're reaching for the sky. Keep your head on the floor. Do your breathing, then hold your breath, suck your stomach up, and go into the exercise position.

DO'S AND DON'TS

- In the exercise position, keep your head tilted back, chin up, so that you don't hurt your neck. Find a spot on the ceiling behind you and focus on that when you are pulling yourself up. In that way, your head will be tilted back in the right position. If you tuck your chin on your chest instead of tilting your head back, you're cheating—you're letting your head and shoulders do all the work instead of your abs, which is what we need the most help with.

- Never rock or push yourself. You want your abs to do the work, not momentum. Imagine you're pulling yourself up by your hands and lowering yourself down again. Don't rest when you hit the ground; keep your abdominal muscles engaged. Just lightly touch the back of your head to the ground before pulling yourself right back up again.

Exercise position: Keeping your arms straight, stretch your hands upward while lifting your shoulders and head off the floor but keeping your head tilted back, looking up at some imaginary point on the ceiling in back of you. Try to get as much of your upper body off the floor as possible. Get your shoulders and chest as high up as you can go. Then roll your body all the way back down so that first the lower back, then the shoulders, and then your head touches the ground. As soon as your head hits the ground, pull yourself all the way back up into the crunch again; keep your head tilted back and arms straight up in the air. Pull yourself up and down to the count of 8 or 10. Do this exercise three times.

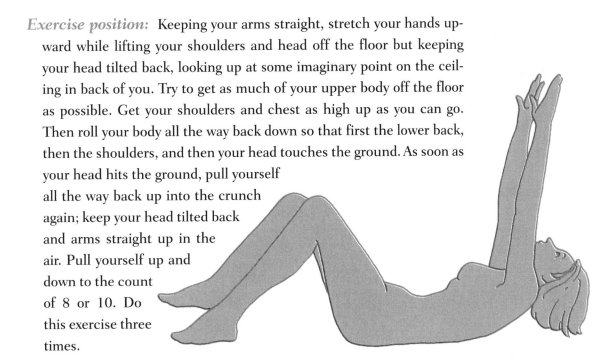

11. THE SCISSORS

This next exercise is for Public Enemy #1, the lower abs.

Starting position: Lie down on the floor with your legs straight and to-gether; point your toes. Take your hands and slip them, palms down, under your rear end so you can support your back. Keep your head on the floor and the small of your back pressed to the floor; this will help protect your back. Do your breathing, suck in your stomach, and hold your breath, then go into the exercise position.

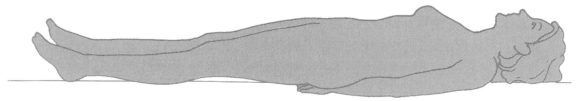

Exercise position: Raise both legs together about 3 or 4 inches off the floor. Making the swipes as wide as you can, begin an over-and-under "scissors" motion, crossing one leg over the other, then under the other, keeping your toes pointed. Swipe over under, over under, over under to the count of 8 or 10. Release your breath. Do three repetitions.

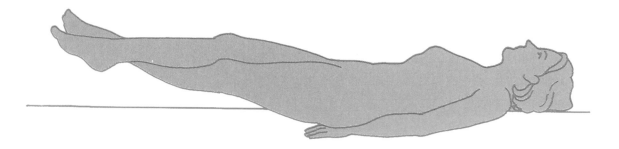

DO'S AND DON'TS

- Remember to keep your palms under your butt and the small of your back pressed to the floor to protect your back. Don't let your back arch.

- Make sure when you do the "scissors" motion that your feet are no more than 3 to 4 inches off the floor—this puts the most stress on your abdomen.

- Always point your toes to put additional stress on the abs and the thighs.

- Don't lift your head off the ground.

- Swipes should be as wide as they can be and be done as fast as you can do them.

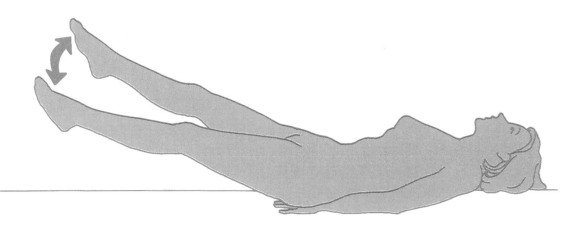

12. THE *C*AT

*T*he Cat is probably the most beneficial exercise of them all because it does the most. It affects the entire abdominal area and the hips. It also helps the back dramatically. The reason that the majority of people have back pain is that they have weak abdominal muscles and the back is doing the work the abdominal muscles should be doing. When you strengthen the abdominal muscles, you take the pressure off the back.

Starting position: Get down on your hands and knees. Your palms should be flat on the floor, arms straight, and back flat. Keep your head up and facing straight ahead. Do the breathing, hold your breath, suck your stomach up, and go into the exercise position.

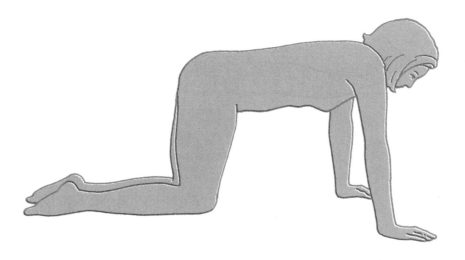

DO'S AND DON'TS

- When done right, this exercise should be one smooth, rolling motion of your body from the stomach through the arching of the back.

Exercise position: Now bow your head; at the same time, pull your back up and arch it as much as possible, stretching your spine so that you look like an angry cat. Hold this arched position to the count of 8 or 10. Release your breath and your back. Repeat this exercise three times.

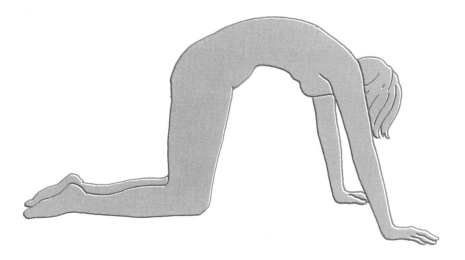

Your Cheat Sheet Chart

Here's a simple chart to help you keep track of the different exercises. You can do them in any order. I like to begin in a standing position, so I start with the two face exercises, the Lion and Ugly Face. That way I warm up with ten deep breaths. Then I go into my Side Stretch before moving to the floor for the rest of the exercises. I always like to finish up with the Cat because it just feels so good.

1. The Lion

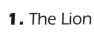 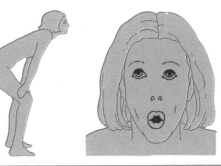 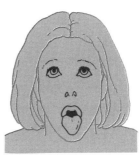

2. The Ugly Face

3. The Side Stretch

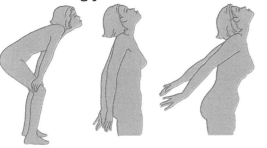 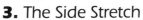 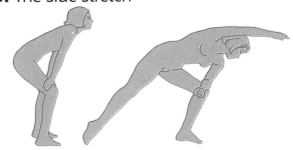

4. The Back Leg Extension

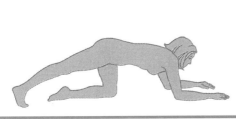

5. The Seiko

6. The Diamond

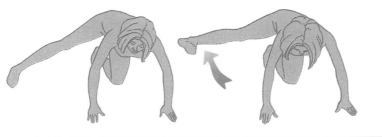 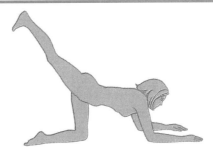 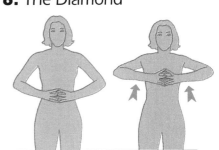

7. The Rowboat

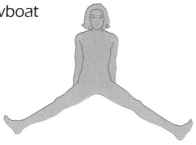 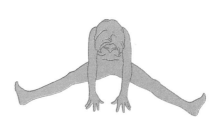

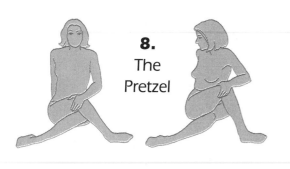

8.
The
Pretzel

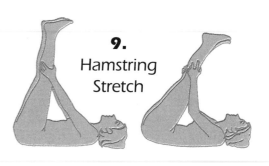

9.
Hamstring
Stretch

10. The Abdominal Crunch

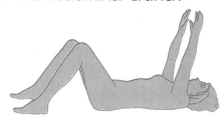

11. The Scissors

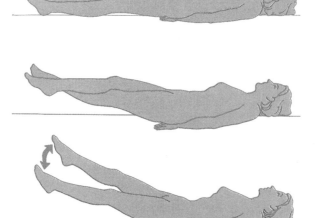

12. The Cat

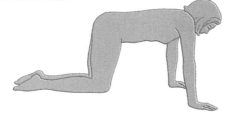

*Y*our Heart's Going Pit-a-Pat
Is it Love or BodyFlex—or Both?

What might you feel when you are doing BodyFlex? When most people first begin this exercise, they find themselves getting hot and perspiring a little bit to moderately. They may also find themselves a little to moderately winded; they may begin coughing a lot, and their hearts may start to beat a little faster. However, everyone's body and chemistry is different, so you can be doing the program correctly and not experience any of these things. If you are experiencing any of the above, you will probably find as time goes on— and it may only be three to four days or a week—that you won't cough anymore, you won't be winded anymore, you won't be light-headed anymore.

But you may still get hot and you may even perspire more because you are getting better at the exercise. Plus, your heart rate will still get up. The reason you want your heart rate to increase during exercise is to pump out the oxygenated blood. But even if you don't get hot or perspire or get your heart rate up, which normally comes from exertion (and recent literature has shown that the heart rate only needs to come up a little during exercise to provide benefit), it doesn't mean that you are doing the program wrong. How do you know when you're doing BodyFlex correctly? You start to lose the inches and you have more energy. It's that simple.

How to Make the BodyFlex Program Fit Your Needs

The beauty of this entire BodyFlex program is that it is simple and uncomplicated. And short. There's one position for each area of the body we need to target. And, yes, we can do what works for us in each position. If you can't do one of the positions to the maximum, do it the best you can. Because we all have to start somewhere.

Let's say, for example, you're going to do the Abdominal Crunch and you have a problem with arthritis in your arms. You don't have to reach your arms to the ceiling. You can cross your arms over your chest (sorry, but the only analogy I can think of is like a dead person) and then you come up and down. You don't have the reaching motion, but you're still stressing the area you want to tone—the abdominals. You can adjust the exercise to what feels right for you as long as the basic position is there. Or let's say you can't come all the way up and go all the way down. Well, maybe you can lift your upper body off the floor 3 or 4 inches for the first few days and 4 or 5 for the next few days and so on.

Or maybe you can't do the Cat because your knees hurt. Well, you can use a cushioned exercise mat if you've got one, but if not, do the exercise on your bed. Do it on a soft surface so you'll have no problems with your knees hurting. You can also do the Back Leg Extension on your bed so you don't hurt your knees and joints. If you're older and you can't lift your leg to the ceiling, lift it 2 or 3 inches off the ground. The truth is that each day and each week you do this program, you'll get stronger and stronger and better and better and more flexible. And as long as you are putting stress on the part of the body you want to tone, you are going to get results—that's if you're doing the breathing, of course. The bottom line is that you can adjust this program and improvise to suit yourself, again, as long as the basic position is still there.

If you're in a wheelchair, you can improvise. If you want to do the Side Stretch, for instance, while seated, take your arm and reach over the top of your head so that you stretch that side area. You can do the breathing and then lean over and reach. Suppose you're sitting in your wheelchair and you want to do an ab exercise. Well, how about if you just do the Scissors? How about if you just put your legs out in front of you and cross over and under and over and under? Even if you've moved from your wheelchair to the bed, you can try to pull yourself a little bit off the bed, even if it's an inch or two. And you're going to get benefit even if you come off the bed an inch, as long as you're doing the breathing.

And that's the point of this exercise. You can work it around and kind of change it a little bit so it's not so hard for you. If you did nothing but the breathing, what you would do is lose excess body fat and increase energy. But the whole idea is that we don't want to be simply a smaller version of what we already are. We want to eliminate the flab on the inside of our legs, get rid of the sagging butt and flabby tummy. So we have to do things to resculpt our bodies, nip a lump here, tighten up the flab here. So we combine the two—body fat loss with inch reduction. And even if the only thing you ever got out of this was more energy, wouldn't you have to say that was worth fifteen minutes a day? The truth is that when you increase oxygen flow to the body, you don't have to wait for results. You have instant energy on the spot.

Have It Your Way

The thing of it is that everybody is different. While I may want to work my legs and butt, somebody else might say, "You know what? My legs and butt look fine. I want to work on my arms and stomach." Another beauty of this program is that you can modify it to your personal problems, whereas if you're on a treadmill or an ab cruncher, that's it.

There is an alternative way to do BodyFlex. For the first five years I taught Bodyflex, I had my clients do spot focusing. On Day One, I'd have them do fifteen minutes of just abs. On Day Two, I'd have them do fifteen minutes of just legs. On Day Three, I'd have them do fifteen minutes of just upper body. And so on. It's very effective, but it's easy to get bored, so watch out.

Ab/waist Workout

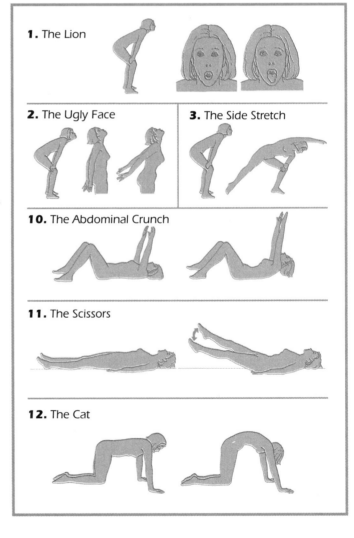

1. The Lion

2. The Ugly Face

3. The Side Stretch

10. The Abdominal Crunch

11. The Scissors

12. The Cat

Thighs/Butt Workout

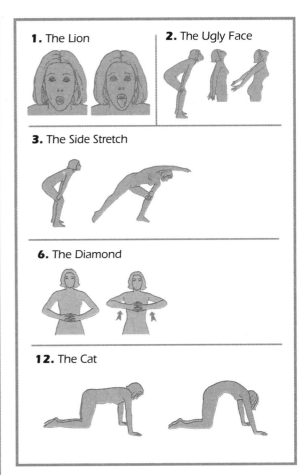

1. The Lion

2. The Ugly Face

8. The Pretzel

9. Hamstring Stretch

4. The Back Leg Extension

5. The Seiko

7. The Rowboat

12. The Cat

Upper Body Workout

1. The Lion

2. The Ugly Face

3. The Side Stretch

6. The Diamond

12. The Cat

Life in the Fast Lane

By the way, you can even do the breathing while driving in the car, although it might be best to do it only when you're in one-lane traffic with the windows up so that no one can pull up beside you and see the expression on your face or hear the sounds of this particular kind of heavy breathing. However, no one to my knowledge has ever been arrested for "obscene driving." You can do arm exercises in the car: suck in your stomach and press your hands on either side of the steering wheel (elbows up, of course), putting a resistance on your upper arms. You can also do the facial exercises (if you're not worried about being carted off to the zoo).

Twice a Day Keeps the Flab Away

I also recommend to people who are first starting this program that they should do it twice a day, in the morning before eating and again in the evening before dinner—if you haven't had anything in your stomach for at least two hours. It jump-starts the results and gets your body used to the increased oxygen in your system. However, watch out for burnout. You want to keep the program easy so you won't ever find an excuse to drop it. If twice a day makes you feel burned-out or resentful, forget it.

BodyFlex is also a great pickup when you're feeling draggy toward late afternoon. If you find yourself feeling tired as the day goes on, close your office door or duck into a restroom stall (if you're not at home) and do about ten breaths. You will feel energized and ready to tackle anything.

Enjoy!

7

Don't Waste Your Breath

Answers to the Most Commonly Asked Questions About BodyFlex

I am very fortunate because I get a lot of feedback and questions from folks who have discovered BodyFlex. And now I want to share with you some of the most frequently asked questions I get about the BodyFlex workout:

- What kind of results can I expect to see in one week? Two weeks? One month? Three months?

I have personally analyzed thousands of measurement charts from the clients to whom I have taught Body-Flex over the last twelve years. I found that the average participant's inch loss after the first week on BodyFlex is somewhere between 4 and 14 inches in their midsection alone. (What I define as your midsection is your waist, hips, thighs, and upper and lower abs. This is the area that women have the biggest problems with.) A lot of the folks I work with come in somewhere between the 8- and 9-inch mark. Some of you will lose more, some less. It's been my experience that people who are already fairly fit to begin with don't lose as dramatically as folks with a lot more to lose. I designed the program based on everything that was wrong with me, figuring if it's wrong with me, it's going to be wrong with every other woman out there. We're all the same, except to different degrees. Most of us have had kids, we're getting older, menopause is setting in, we're starting to gain weight in our hips and our rear—it's the same story for all of us.

One thing I can't predict is how much you are going to lose and where. I can assure you if you do it right, you'll lose. But after about three to four weeks on any program, not just BodyFlex, people plateau. You can expect to plateau for about five to seven days, then you'll start dropping inches again. It's a normal process for all fitness programs and this is no exception. People will call me because they've had dramatic inch loss in one week, two weeks, three weeks, then all of a sudden they stop. I assure them that they are just at a plateau, but that they're going to kick back out and start losing inches again. Then after about four or five more weeks, you'll plateau again for maybe about a week. It's a normal process with all exercise. Always remember: Plateaus are part of the process. Don't freak out when you hit one and give up the program. I know it's frustrating to keep working away and not see the results, but fight the temptation to quit. Stay with it, and you'll see more results again soon.

If you're doing BodyFlex to get more energy, you won't have to wait for results. The good news with BodyFlex is that when it comes to energy, it's just like driving your car. When you put gas in your car, you don't have to wait for the car to perform—it starts right up and takes off. That's just the way the body responds with body fuel—oxygen. When you incorporate more body fuel, your body will instantly perform. You should see a difference in the first twenty-four hours with this program. You will feel more energized, stronger, more vibrant, more relaxed. You will feel like a healthier person in the first twenty-four hours.

■ If I want quicker results, should I do more reps or hold the positions longer?

I tell most people out there: Don't overdo it, you're going to burn yourself out. When you start seeing yourself getting great results, you start thinking, "Oh boy, if one is good then two is better. If five seconds is good, then twenty seconds is better." The thing of it is, I want you in this for the long haul, and I think you want yourself in it for the long haul. So if you're in it for the long haul, you have to make it doable and easy. Otherwise, you're outta there.

So my recommendation is this: For the first week and the first week only, you can do this program twice a day, once before breakfast, once before dinner. Or you can do it back-to-back before breakfast or back-to-back before dinner, whenever your stomach is empty. This allows your metabolism to get a jump-start. Many of you out there reading this have had a low metabolism for so long that it's going to take more than fifteen minutes a day the first week to get this thing jacked up.

But only double your workout for the first week, because fifteen minutes a day is very doable and palatable. Trust me: After about a month or so, when you start looking at doing it twice a day, you're going to start not looking forward to doing it. Then you're going to find reasons not to do it, and before you know it, you're going to stop doing it. Fifteen minutes is just the right amount of time that you can do it and not get tired of it and think it's too much. You'd have a pretty difficult time explaining to yourself, as you look in the mirror, that you don't have fifteen minutes for yourself in a day. As I mentioned in the last chapter, you don't want to burn out by doing it too much. It's pretty hard to make an excuse not to do BodyFlex.

You can hold your breath in each position for up to a count of 12, but you don't need to go any higher to get optimum results. I usually tell my clients to aim for a count of 8 to 10.

- What do I do if my nose is stuffed up and I can't breathe through it? Can I still do BodyFlex?

A lot of my clients have sinus problems, deviated septums, allergies, all kind of nasal problems that make them stuffed up. I tell them to go into the bathroom first thing in the morning, because that's when their noses are the most stuffed up, and turn the hot shower on, close the door, and leave for a moment. Then I tell them to go back in when the bathroom is full of steam and to shut the door and do about five of the BodyFlex breaths—just the breathing part, from blowing out to the abdominal lift. It should help clear the sinuses.

It's okay to miss the BodyFlex workout for one or two days, but really try to get back on track as soon as you can. If you don't do BodyFlex for a week or two, you're going to start going back to what you were. Even if you're not up to the full fifteen minutes, do what you can to stay on the program.

- What if I'm not seeing results?

If you have been doing this program religiously for seven days and you see no results, it could be because you're not doing the technique right. Review the steps in Chapter 5 and practice the technique again. Or perhaps you're one of the millions who are on thyroid medication, birth control medication, antidepressants, or have an extremely low metabolism. If that is the case, *do not* get discouraged. I started working with a client who was a size 22. And I thought, isn't she going to be great? She's a perfect example and she's going to lose so fast, and I know she was doing the program right because I was personally teaching her every single day. The first two weeks, the woman lost nothing, not one inch. And I thought, what in the world? But after the second week going into the third week, her measurements just started to plummet.

I can't tell you exactly why it takes some people longer than others to see results. My average client, in the first seven days, lost 4 to 14 inches. But there are always going to be exceptions. There are always going to be people who won't see results in the first week. Don't panic. Keep going. Because if you don't see results the first week, you'll probably see them the second week. And if you don't get results the second week, keep on going. I don't think I've ever had a client who hadn't gotten results after three weeks.

As with any fitness program, especially one this unique and different, you're going to have some questions. "Am I doing this right?" is the main thing people ask me. This is one of the programs where the more you do it, the better you get. It's just a matter of practice because, let's face it, it's a very odd technique. And you'll find you'll be working areas you have never worked before, such as the stomach and other internal organs. This is the only technique I've ever seen that stimulates, and exercises, the organs in the body, getting them to work at a higher rate of efficiency. When you do this exercise, the stomach, pancreas, and liver get pulled in and rolled up and massaged, so to speak. Many people have reported fewer digestive problems when they do BodyFlex. Again, if you're doing the exercises right, during the last stage, which is the abdominal lift, your stomach will actually be concave. I call this working the muscles from the inside out rather than the outside in.

If you're losing inches and feeling more energetic, you're doing BodyFlex correctly. But listen to your body's other signs, too. If you can go up a flight of stairs without feeling winded or your digestive system isn't giving you as much trouble, it probably means you're in the BodyFlex groove.

You'll also know that you're doing BodyFlex right if you've got more endurance and stamina while you're doing the workout. You don't feel light-headed anymore. You can hold for a count of 8 or 10—or even longer—without any trouble. And you'll be able to do Step 3—the forceful exhalation of air—from deep down in the diaphragm. You'll be able to hear the difference.

- How can I combine BodyFlex with other workouts?

I designed BodyFlex to be a workout all by itself. It's a complete aerobic workout in just fifteen minutes. So I tell people, yes, you can combine it with other workouts. But why would you want to? We are all on such a time crunch that we barely have fifteen minutes, let alone time for some other regimen. BodyFlex will improve your flexibility, cardiovascular fitness, and muscle tone.

But if you've got the time and the ambition, I say go for it, and good for you. Just do your BodyFlex first so you won't be tempted to blow it off. And try to resist trading off BodyFlex with other exercise, because you might find yourself slipping out of your fifteen-minute routine. If you're lucky enough to have an hour for a game of tennis or a brisk walk, please squeeze in that extra fifteen minutes for BodyFlex. It will improve your stamina for tennis, running, walking, and other physical endeavors.

However, as we women get older, we need to be more concerned about strong bones as well as flexibility, and for that we need weight-bearing exercises beyond BodyFlex. I'll discuss those options in the next chapter.

> ■ How come all the health magazines say I can't "spot reduce," but you say I can direct oxygen to specific parts of my body?

Many health magazines and health authorities say it is impossible to spot reduce. But they've been wrong about a lot of things before, and I think they're wrong on this point, too. If you can spot build, which is what bodybuilders do all the time, why can't you spot reduce? They can put any name they want on it, but when someone can lose 4 to 14 inches in their midsection in one week, I call that "spot reduction." A bodybuilder will use weights to specifically work his biceps, for example, because he wants to build them up. That's spot building. You spot reduce the opposite way. Instead of using weights to build up the muscle, you use stretches to elongate the muscle. That produces inch loss in a particular area. And inch loss in a designated area is by definition spot reduction.

We have learned that blood is the transportation system for oxygen and that the only thing that burns fat in the body is oxygen. So what we need to do is get more oxygen to the body, by aerobic breathing, then get it traveling around in the body to our fattest areas. We have to put a stress on the fat areas with isometric, isotonic, or stretch positions to direct the oxygenated blood there. Anytime we put stress or a stretch on a particular area, it creates a need for more blood, which is carrying the oxygen, which burns the fat in that area. If that's not spot reducing, I don't know what is.

> ■ I just spent months at the "butt busters" class and aerobic dance classes at my local gym and now my legs are actually bigger than when I started! How do I know this won't happen with BodyFlex?

A common mistake most women make is that we get motivated, then we're off to the races before we even understand what we're doing. We see somebody on TV or in a magazine or a movie and we want to look like her. Before we even have the proper information, we run to the gym and start exercising and lifting weights and working out on machines. We think we're on the right track. The problem is after three months of doing all these things, we look down and see our legs are getting bigger. The bigger problem is that we don't understand what aerobic exercise is— we think it means strenuous activity or movement.

Again, the aerobic part of all activity is in the breathing, not the activity. And aerobic breathing is what burns fat. What is happening at your typical aerobic dance class is that you are not breathing deeply enough in an aerobic way to burn off body fat. So you are simply building muscle under existing fat, particularly in the leg area because that's the area you're putting the most stress or stretch on when you're hopping up and down and on and off your step platform. And yes, your legs are getting toned up but they are getting bigger and bulkier at the same time. Again, the ticket is to burn off the body fat through breathing exercises while simultaneously toning muscle so that you can see the most defined muscle underneath.

- Can deep breathing help break down cellulite?

Yes. Cellulite is simply deposits of fat with metabolic waste material, and that waste material makes it hard for the blood to get to the area when you are breathing normally. Increased circulation through aerobic breathing directed to the area through isometric or isotonic positions will help burn cellulite on the spot. Cellulite normally starts forming on women in the hamstring area first, then slowly moves around the body. The reason it forms in the hamstrings first is because, unless you are a runner, the hamstring muscles don't get stretched that much. Therefore, increasing oxygenated blood to the stagnant area will help burn fat on a cellular level for people affected with cellulite.

- What should I do if I fall off the BodyFlex wagon? How can I stay motivated?

Everyone falls off the wagon, including me. You look at some of these fitness people and you think to yourself, Oh, they've always looked like that. Or they exercise ten times a day. But I've got to tell you that, after all these years, I still fall off the BodyFlex wagon. I want to grab a few extra minutes lazing in bed, or I want to shoot right out of the house to get started on my day. Do you know how I stay motivated? The same way I told you. In the morning, I get up, I go to the bathroom, I take off my nightgown and look at myself front and back, and I say to myself, "I've got to get back on BodyFlex today, I don't have any time to waste." You don't want those lost inches to come back. Looking at yourself in the mirror is remotivation enough for 99 percent of us.

Think about your energy level. It's kind of like being poor. You don't always know just how poor you are when you're poor; it's only when you become rich that you realize how poor you were. It's kind of like that with BodyFlex. You don't realize how bad you were feeling until you feel great. We just get used to dragging around tired and making excuses for ourselves, saying we've got kids and husbands and jobs; no wonder we're tired. But the fact is, we're not all tired. Those doing BodyFlex aren't. And we don't know we feel so crummy until the veil of tiredness is pulled off and we're full of energy. We're tasting the good life for once— vibrancy, energy, get-up-and-go, motivation. Then we know how bad we once felt. I know you don't want to go back to feeling that way. Let your love of being a high-energy person motivate you to stay on track.

Want to be a loser again? Here's another way to motivate yourself. Besides looking at yourself in the mirror, take that pair of pants that didn't fit you before you started BodyFlex. Remember how I told you to keep them around and try them on every week to see how big they were getting on you? Now, remember how loose they had gotten on you before you had fallen off the wagon? If you stop doing the program and you try them on each week again, you'll find they've gotten tighter and tighter and tighter. That should motivate you! If you're losing, keep doing what works and get back in the saddle.

- Why is BodyFlex the best exercise for us as we get older?

As we age, gravity takes over and is ruthless with our bodies. Everything gets pulled down, inside and out, leaving us with saggy, flabby frames. What's the answer? *Prevention* magazine attributes youthfulness to oxygenation and flexibility. But when we do an impact exercise, which means leaving the ground as in jogging or jumping, we affect every joint, from our ankles all the way through our back, when our feet meet the ground again. This jolting helps gravity pull everything down even more. Plus, running, jogging, and the like are not designed to correct a saggy butt or flabby stomach. A nonimpact exercise like BodyFlex is the best, in my opinion, in all ways. Nonimpact exercise doesn't bring on any deterioration of muscle tone. Plus, deep breathing is at the base of all exercise programs, increasing oxygen to the blood to provide the fat-burning we need in a safe technique that really helps save our joints. Simple stretch positions, combined with deep breathing, give you all the flexibility you need as you get older because they elongate muscle.

- How can my metabolism change through Body-Flex?

The whole idea of exercise is just to become aerobic, which means increasing oxygen to the blood through breathing. We then want to direct the blood to the areas we want to affect. The ticket is that you don't need to kill yourself to become aerobic. You need to increase circulation and pump up your lungs and heart and the muscles around your heart.

Speeding up metabolism is about exerting the body enough so that you will huff and puff and breathe more deeply and heavily, thereby increasing oxygen to the blood and giving you more fat-burning ability. When our metabolism is high, our bodies can process food faster. It breaks down faster and doesn't stay in the body as long. When you do aerobic exercise day after day, your metabolism becomes a little higher each day. If you continue to exercise, it will stay high. BodyFlex will help boost your metabolism and keep it boosted.

8

Beyond BodyFlex

*T*here *is* life after BodyFlex.

In fact, you can extend the benefits of this program by taking better care of yourself. Body-Flex itself will be a big part of your desire to do that because it gives you an overall feeling of well-being and tremendous pride in your appearance, and that can inspire you to take additional steps to keep yourself fit.

*S*hould *You Dip in Your Toe or Dive in?*

Before I started BodyFlex, I just didn't care about taking care of myself. I thought the same thing everybody reading this book thinks, What's the difference? I'm overweight, out of shape, who cares if I eat the right things? I'm still not going to look right. So forget it, I'll just keep on living the same old way and I'll figure something else out down the line.

Even when I started BodyFlex, I didn't start eating properly right away because I didn't think the program was going to work. I figured that I wasn't going to give this my all because the 195 other things I had tried before hadn't worked. But I was willing to stick my toe in the water. So I just kept eating the same old way but I got results anyway. And when I saw that 10½-inch loss the first week, I got so excited. And I thought to myself, if I'm eating wrong and doing all the wrong things and I'm losing anyway, I wonder what would happen if I were eating the right way? I wonder how much more I'd be able to lose; I wonder how much better I'd feel? I decided to just check it out. I told myself that I didn't have to keep doing it, but I was going to try it, just to see. And if it didn't work—and it probably wouldn't—then I was going to go back to the same old way of doing things.

So I stopped eating late at night. I used to eat late at night all the time. At nine or ten o'clock, or maybe later, I'd sit down and have a big meal. I made up my mind that after 4:30 in the afternoon, I was not going to eat anything except maybe some salad or something light like that. I began my new eating regimen on the second week of the BodyFlex program. And I dropped down an amazing 14 inches that week. That brought my total inch loss to 24 inches, which averaged out to a foot a week.

BodyFlex worked for me even better the second week than it did the first week because I was eating differently. And not only that, but I was feeling better. I became like those mice that are programmed to run through the maze to get the reward at the end—when they find the right path, they keep running down it to get the reward at the end. I kept doing what I was doing. It's operant conditioning: When we see results, we want to keep repeating the behavior that brings the reward. And the truth is that, with weight and inch loss, all we need to give ourselves the motivation to keep going is to be able to see just a little bit of difference in our bodies; we don't need to see a whole lot of difference. However, with the results I was experiencing, I went from putting my toe in the water to putting in my whole foot.

After that, I started doing a few more of the right things, though not all. I almost *totally* stopped eating at night, number one. I stopped eating many typical American foods: macaroni and cheese, white bread, sweets, red meat, and soda pop. I started incorporating more steamed vegetables into my diet and started cutting out some of the refined carbohydrates.

I learned that carbohydrates feed your energy system. We break down carbohydrates into glucose to run our engines. But refined carbs, like potato chips, candy, ice cream, and simple sugars, go into the motor too quickly and overheat it. The energy burst hits you all at once because all the fiber has been processed out of the food, and fiber is the key to how quickly something is burned in the system. Complex carbohydrates, such as baked potatoes, grains, whole-grain pasta and bread, oatmeal, popcorn, and barley have lots of fiber, and they help the body release energy at a steady rate. So I made an effort to eat less refined, over-processed food, and more natural food high in fiber.

I knew I should have less fat in my diet, so I cut down on butter, but just a little. I didn't do a big dramatic deal; I did all these things just a little bit. But I started feeling a whole lot better and I started getting better results. Something was really happening to my body and I liked what I saw and felt.

So I continued, and pretty soon I started actively looking for things to do that would be even better. Even today, I continue to look for things that are going to be better and better and better for me, to add to my healthy lifestyle and make me feel even better. I read articles, I talk to nutrition experts, I make it my business to find out what's right for me. We can never do too many right things for ourselves. We can do too many wrong things, but we can't do too many right things.

My co-author, Bobbie Katz, had a totally different experience with this program, approaching it almost from the opposite direction. Instead of dipping her toes into altering her diet, she dove in headfirst with a radical change. In her forties, she is one of those people who is on medication for hypothyroidism (low thyroid) and in 1995, her 5 foot 3 inch body had ballooned up to 158 pounds and was fitting, tightly I might add, into a size 12–14. The last time she had been to the doctor, six months before, she had weighed 152 pounds. At that point, disgusted and depressed because nothing was working to get her weight off, she decided to try cutting drastically down on fat, though she did nothing about the portions of food she was consuming. Because she thought she was eating virtually fat-free, she mistakenly thought that she could eat as much as she wanted.

About two weeks before she want back to the doctor, she began the BodyFlex program. While she lost some inches, her initial results were lower than average because of her thyroid problem and the medication. On top of that, when she went into the office to get weighed, unbeknownst to her, she had gained another 6 pounds over the last six months and now weighed 158. Frantic because she was trying to be so careful with her diet and was now exercising as well, she broke down and cried in the doctor's office. The doctor asked her if she was ready to try something drastic to see if her medication was functioning properly (as opposed to her mouth) and she told him that she was. He put her on a 1,000-calorie-a-day diet for two weeks, one that utilized a liquid nutrient at breakfast and lunch and then a little chicken or fish with some vegetables or fresh fruit for dinner. She lost 11 pounds in two weeks. Thinking that diet was all there was to it, she, being like everyone else who doesn't like to exercise, stopped doing BodyFlex, deciding to stay on a low-fat, sugar-free 1,000 calories a day instead.

Excited about her weight loss, Bobbie went into one of the local department stores and tried on a pair of stretch jeans. If she lay down on the floor of the dressing room, she was barely able to squeeze into a size 9, though she took a lot of the skin off her fingers trying to get the zipper up. Still, they were on . . . and they looked good. She figured she'd lose a couple more pounds, then come back and buy the jeans when she could put them on standing up. Another week of calorie deprivation ought to do it. She put a little mark on the tag so that she would be able to identify which pair she had poured herself into and happily went home.

The following week, still on her 1,000-calorie-a-day diet, she discovered that she had lost another five pounds. Really excited now, she went back to the department store to find the pair of jeans she had tried on the week before, thinking she could now get the zipper up with little effort. Finding them at the bottom of the pile where she had "hidden" them, she ran into the dressing room to try them on. Imagine her surprise when she couldn't even get them up over her thighs. She had lost five more pounds but somehow she was bigger. It was then she realized that she might have been losing weight, but it was BodyFlex that was responsible for her inch loss and for contouring her body.

Bobbie started the BodyFlex program again and has done it every day since. She went from a size 12–14 to a size 1–3, where she remains today, within three months. And, yes, now she is eating very healthily. No more artificial liquid diets. Just a lot of fruits and vegetables, with some chicken and fish. Proud of her appearance for the first time in years, and motivated into keeping herself looking as good and feeling as good as she does, she, too, is trying to do as many right things for herself as she can. And, by the way, where do you think she got the energy to write this book while doing her regular work as well? From BodyFlex, of course!

I think the bottom line of all fitness programs is to get in shape and stay that way and still be able to live a normal life in the process. I think eating is one of the joys of living and that we can't ask ourselves to give up too much. We simply want to modify what we're doing so that we can live a normal life and lose and be fit anyway. The problem with most diets is that they ask people to sacrifice more than they can handle. People aren't rabbits; they can't be satisfied eating a couple of leaves of lettuce and a few carrot sticks. As I said, the main thing I preach about Body-Flex is that you can live a normal life and basically eat the way you want to and still be fit. You just have to be conscious of a few basics.

It's All in the Timing

When it comes to food, the time of day you eat has a lot to do with what's going to happen to you weight-wise. When your metabolism is up, you can eat more. You can eat more frequently and you can eat more volume because your raised metabolic rate speeds up the processing of your food so that you can burn it off. The Europeans have it down the right way. They eat a huge breakfast, a middle-sized lunch, and a little tiny dinner. Here, in America, we do it the opposite. We eat little or no breakfast, we eat a middle-sized lunch, and then, at eight or nine o'clock at night, when our metabolism is very low, we eat our biggest meal. Then we go from the dining table to the sofa and the rest is history. BIG history. I tell my clients that if they don't eat after 4:30 or 5:00 in the afternoon, they are going to be in pretty good shape. That's not very realistic for all of us, but the point is that the earlier—and lighter—the dinner, the better.

If you can't eat your last meal of the day in the late afternoon, try this instead: Have a healthy snack late in the afternoon, so you won't be starving when it's dinnertime, and you'll be able to eat a very light meal and feel satisfied. I love to snack on raw almonds (a great source of protein), organic raisins, popcorn (lots of fiber but go easy on the salt), or my "green" drink (see page 162). Don't have a heavy meal before you go to bed because it's too hard on the digestive system—as I've said, nighttime is when your metabolism is at its slowest.

Whenever I snack, I try to go organic. Organic food is full of nutrition, alkaline minerals (which the body needs to maintain its normal pH), and vitamins. When food is processed, it is depleted of all these things. Plus, when plants are grown on nonorganic farms, they are grown several times on the same soil. Eventually the nutrients are depleted from the soil. If they're not in the soil, they're not in the plants.

Go Halfsies

I tell people that there are two things they can do to get themselves in shape and stay in shape. One is to reduce sugar in the diet by half and the other is to reduce salt in the diet by half. If you can do these two things and keep doing exactly what you're doing now, then you're going to lose weight and be a heck of a lot healthier.

One-half of a nonfat bagel, which you might think is a healthy way to eat, breaks down to one-third cup of pure sugar in your system. And besides making you fat, sugar robs your body of nutrients. I think sugar and salt are the body's biggest enemies, responsible in part for such ailments as headaches, constipation, and irritable bowel syndrome.

Today's emphasis on a diet high in complex carbohydrates doesn't support good health, especially if it doesn't include enough vegetables. Refined carbs, including soda, processed breakfast cereals, and alcohol, greatly stress the metabolic process, often resulting in hypoglycemic distress. As I mentioned, refined carbs produce energy in great bursts, taxing the body's ability to regulate energy. Ultimately, this causes a lack of energy; after a few years, a person can become burned out and absolutely dependent on quick energy fixes from sugar, coffee, and so on.

Carbs, like protein, leave an acidic waste in the body. And most diseases, including cancer, are acidic in nature. Therefore, whenever you eat a complex carb meal, you should also have vegetables and salad so that the alkaline minerals from the vegetables can buffer the acidic residue.

You may have noticed that you feel sleepy after a big meal of complex carbohydrates. That's because complex carbs cause a release of hormones that promotes drowsiness. Therefore, you might want to consume your complex carbs at the last meal of the day.

As for salt, it's not that it's bad—it is essential in the diet—but that we're getting way too much in our diets. The average person needs only 250 milligrams a day, yet takes in between 4,000 to 10,000 milligrams per day. And only 15 percent of that is from the salt shaker. The rest comes from processed foods (check the label; anything with the word *sodium* contains salt).

Salt can inhibit the digestive enzymes so they can't break down food properly. Salt also causes the body to retain water, making you feel bloated. It also keeps you from eliminating waste effectively because the salt binds with the waste. Salt is associated with high blood pressure in some people.

If you reduce your salt consumption gradually, you'll find that you'll reduce the craving from your "salt tooth." Try using natural flavorings such as lemon and herbs instead.

*T**here's that F Word Again*

What about fat? You cannot be healthy without the proper fats in your system, but there are fats that kill and fats that heal. Essential fatty acids are those that cannot be produced by the body; they must come from a dietary source. They are good fats as opposed to bad fats, which are processed nonessential (hydrogenated) fats that solidify in the bloodstream and clog arteries. Good fats can help keep the metabolic rate higher. The essential fats in the liver allow the amino acids from protein to be utilized by the body. Our nerves are covered by a myelin sheath, which is composed of essential fatty acids. This covering insulates the nerves almost like duct tape around a live wire.

Essential fats are found in such foods as cold water fish, wild game (pheasant, deer), organic eggs, flaxseed oil, pumpkin seed oil, soya, olives, seeds, and nuts. Human breast milk is full of these fats, allowing a baby to develop his nervous system among many other functions, while cow's milk doesn't have these essential fatty acids. Processed or nonessential fats are found in such items as corn oil, vegetable oil, margarine, potato chips, cookies, etc. These are the fats that kill.

Besides allowing the body to utilize protein, essential fats raise the HDL or good cholesterol, lubricate the skin, and help prevent damage to the nervous system. I take two tablespoons of flaxseed oil myself daily—it's one of those essential fats the body needs and is also vital to the suppleness of your skin. I'll take some flaxseed oil, some juice from a fresh lemon, some garlic, and a little pepper and make a dressing for salads. It tastes wonderful and it's very good for you.

In general, though, where fat in the diet is concerned, I don't go down the same road as conventional thinkers. The problem with most people is that at one meal they're talking about fat grams, at the next meal they're talking about carbohydrates, at the next meal they're talking about something else. I don't know about you, but I can't follow any kind of diet plan unless it's consistent all the way through. The plan I promote is that if you make vegetables—raw or steamed—60 percent of your diet, it doesn't matter what you do with the other 40 percent.

Veggies to the Rescue

Actually, the healthiest breakfast you could eat would be a plate of fresh spinach with some carrots and cucumbers and a little bit of low-fat dressing, because greens and vegetables feed the cells in the body. It's not so much that you are what you eat, but that you are what you can absorb. And vegetables (raw or steamed), besides providing the highest content of fiber, vitamins, minerals, and micronutrients, also provide the enzymes the body needs to break down the food we eat.

As I mentioned, vegetables buffer everything else you eat. And there's all kinds of things you can make with them that are delicious and that fill you up. Most important, vegetables produce and provide all the micronutrients the body needs, and they are the foods that are the highest in fiber.

The good news is that having a lot of fiber in your system helps you get rid of anything else that you eat that may not be so good for you. Normally when you eat something that contains fat, it stays in the system because your diet does not have enough fiber in it to move it out. So it is reabsorbed into your system and makes you fat. However, when your diet contains 60 percent vegetables, the fiber in the vegetables helps move the fat through so it is more quickly processed through the system and eliminated.

Experts at the American Cancer Society and the American Heart Association tell us that we should be eating between five and nine servings of fruit and vegetables a day. Did you know that for optimum health, some nutrition experts recommend you should be eating fifteen *pounds* of raw vegetables a day? Of course, that's impossible, but it gives you an indication of how important vegetables and greens are to our diet.

Fruit is very cleansing to the body. Disease is most often caused by one of two things: toxicity or deficiency. When the body is toxic, fruit will help cleanse it. Fruit is easy to digest and full of vitamins, minerals, and enzymes. If you have a late-night meal heavy in complex carbohydrates, you should have fruit the next morning for break-fast. But I wouldn't have just fruit in the morning instead of vegetables and protein plus essential oils. That won't give you the energy you need.

I recommend eating fruit as an in-between-meal snack and only when it is in season and at the height of its freshness so that you get all the vitamins and minerals. Eat fruit alone, never with protein, carbs, or fats, as fruit requires much less time to be digested and in combination with these foods can cause gastic distress. I'd also avoid fruit juices like the plague. They are way too high in sugar. When in nature would you sit and eat five oranges? That's what you have in a cup of orange juice—five oranges, five tablespoons of sugar, and *no* fiber.

Sources of Protein	Sources of Refined Carbs	Sources of Complex Carbs	Sources of Essential Fats	Sources of Processed Fats
Eggs	White refined breads	**Vegetables that are high in complex carbs:** carrots, lentils, pumpkin, beans (boiled), potatoes, rutabaga, Jerusalem artichoke	Cold-water fish	Corn oil
Cold-water fish	Cookies		Wild game	Vegetable oil
Seeds and nuts	Pies		Organic eggs	Butter
Turkey	Sugar		Flaxseed oil	Margarine
Chicken	Crackers		Pumpkin seed oil	Mayonnaise
Wild game	Syrup		Soya	Potato chips
Shellfish	Cakes		Olives	Cookies, etc.
Dairy	Candy		Seeds and nuts	
Beans	Bottled fruit juice	**Cereals and grains:** Rice, spelt, wheat, oatmeal, popcorn, corn, buckwheat, barley, millet, granola, quinoa, rye meal, grits, hominy, whole-grain breads		
Red meat	Chewing gum			
Tofu	Refined pasta			

Meat Makes Me See Red

An interesting fact is that the only time animals get cancer is when they are domesticated and people feed them table scraps. Animals in the wild don't get cancer because they don't eat cooked food. They get all their nutrients from the raw foods in nature. I worry that some of those hormones used to raise our meat today might end up inside of you when you cook and eat meat. Animals in the wild eat raw meat. The whole key to health is that the more man touches it, the less you want it. Plus, cooked food is hard to digest.

I hardly ever eat red meat. I eat chicken twice a week and fish once a week. I eat a lot of tofu for protein. You can eat it in all different ways, even in salad dressing and pudding.

Red meat has been associated with the development of colon cancer. And we know meat is pure protein so it is very difficult to digest; remember how you feel after you've downed a big steak or hamburger? That means you are going to have a lot of waste in your system. If you have any problem with constipation, these toxins just lie in the system and are reabsorbed. We need a clean, clear system to have everything working the right way. So I'd cut down your red meat consumption or give it up altogether.

Mom Was Right: Chew Your Food

Sixty percent of all digestion takes place in the mouth. The other 40 percent takes place from the stomach and colon down. Everybody thinks food goes down into the digestive tract and away it goes. When you start chewing your food, it triggers the digestive enzymes to start breaking down the food. You should chew your food really well so that it's almost like a liquid before you swallow it. That really aids in the digestive process, which will help keep your system cleared out.

The problem most of us have is that we are always in a hurry, so we eat very fast. We don't chew our food, and when we don't chew our food, our digestive system really has a double-duty overtime job to do. A lot of our food doesn't get digested properly, or at all, if it is not chewed properly. Plus, if the food is not digested as it's going down, it's going to just fly through the system and come out without delivering any nutrients to our bodies. Eighty percent of the absorption of minerals and nutrients takes place in the colon. That's why doctors tell people to use suppositories when they want something to get into the system fast—it is absorbed very quickly and goes right into the bloodstream.

So listen to your mom for once and chew your food. When you eat slowly, you also get to really enjoy what you're eating. Ever have the experience of getting up from the table with no memory of having eaten? Why deprive yourself of the joy of your meals? Make mealtime a relaxing time.

The Incredible Shrinking Stomach

I've been saying for many years that volume, or the amount of food you eat, has nothing to do with the effectiveness of BodyFlex. The truth is that, after four, five days of being on this program, your stomach starts to contract because you're working the stomach and the muscles around it. Your stomach gets smaller and you can't put as much food in it. So when you start to eat, you fill up faster. I used to ask all my classes, after the first week, how many of them couldn't eat as much at one sitting? They all raised their hands. Then I asked how many of them filled up faster when they put the same amount of food on their plates that they had always had and they all raised their hands again. What happens is your stomach contracts, your appetite naturally starts to reduce, and you don't consume as much food. That fact alone is going to help you lose body fat. That's why I advise my classes not to worry about counting calories or fat grams. Just stop eating when you feel full. Don't go on automatic pilot and polish off everything on your plate because it's there and you want to be in the "Clean Plate Club." Listen to your body's signals that it's full and put your fork down.

One from Column A and One from Column B

I know the experts disagree with one another on this, but I also really approve of food-combining. Now I know it's hard, and you're probably thinking, Shoot, I work all day long and I come home and can't be worrying about what foods should be eaten with what. But a good rule of thumb to follow to make it real simple—and I believe in simplicity—is that you never eat protein and carbohydrate together at one sitting. You can have protein and carbohydrate during the day, you just can't have them together at the same meal.

When you have a protein, say, meat, and a carbohydrate, like potatoes, what happens is that it doesn't break down properly in your system. So it's more likely to get turned into fat. That's because you only have one stomach and it takes hydrochloric acid in your system to break down protein and an alkaline base to break down complex carbohydrates like potatoes. The alkaline neutralizes the acid, so nothing gets processed. The enzymes used to digest protein are more costly to the body to manufacture than the ones that break down carbohydrates, so if you eat protein and carbs simultaneously, the body may only respond with the easier carbohydrate digestive process and let more of the protein pass through undigested. This results in poor absorption, which stresses the system. When you have protein, you should have vegetables or salad with it because it doesn't require any strong stuff to break them down.

Get Juiced

As I said before, the best thing in the whole wide world that people can have in their system is greens. So a good thing to have in the morning is a "green" drink. Everyone should own a blender or a juicer. This is what I do in the morning: I take two handfuls of alfalfa sprouts and throw them into a blender. I then take one banana, half a cup of water, half a cup of organic apple juice, and one scoop of barley green and put them in the blender as well. I turn the blender on and let it go. When I'm done, I've got a nutritional drink that is like a full breakfast. And sprouts . . . you can't even imagine how healthy they are for your body. This drink is healthy, full of nutrition, and tastes great.

Get Wet

I also recommend drinking eight glasses of water a day. I recommend you drink them with lemon because lemon is a natural diuretic that helps cleanse the organs. Water, on its own, helps flush out the system and rid it of toxins and fat. It has been proven that water helps expedite the results of all fitness programs, not just this one. If you drink mineral or spring water, make sure it is noncarbonated. I'd also avoid sugary soda.

Once we find something that works for us, such as BodyFlex, we get real excited because we've been disappointed so many times. We want to keep looking as good and feeling as good as possible. So we naturally want to do the things that are healthiest and most beneficial for us. And, as I said before, there are some things we can do without sacrificing too much and have a much healthier lifestyle. We can still get lots to eat—and we all love to eat—and be in much better condition. To me, it's what you do 80 percent of the time that really counts. Nobody's going to be perfect and adhere to a perfect diet all the time. But if 80 percent of the time you do the right things, you're going to be in good shape—look good, feel good, be healthier, and have much less chance of something going wrong with your body.

Save Your Skeleton

Along with eating well, there is something else you can do to keep your bones strong. I believe in doing the least amount possible and getting the most results from it—like most other people, I don't want to do anything at all. So for seventeen years, all I've ever done is BodyFlex because it's all I've ever needed. Now I'm in my fifties and I'm going through the change of life. My doctor said to me, "Greer, you need to do some kind of strength training." And I said to him, "What does that mean?" He explained that when you enter perimenopause and then menopause itself, your bones start to deteriorate at a rate of 10 percent a year. They become frail and brittle, and if you fall, you can easily break a hip. You're a sitting duck for osteoporosis. We need to keep our bones strong so that we can stay agile and have a full range of movement as well as being able to look and feel as young as we possibly can. What you need to do to maintain bone density—and it starts deteriorating fast—is some sort of strength training, exercise that puts direct stress on the bones, forcing them to become stronger. Resistance training is a type of strength training. In resistance training, you put a resistance, or stress, on the body with a heavy elastic band or free weight beyond what it can normally tolerate. This causes the body to adapt to the additional stress and become stronger.

Many doctors recommend lifting free weights to help build up bones. I'm not talking about bench-pressing like Arnold. I'm talking about lifting light one- or two-pound weights. Studies have been done on women in nursing homes, and the results showed that weight lifting even helped women in their eighties and nineties strengthen their bones. Ask your doctor if weight training would work for you.

I've got to be honest; although I know it can be effective for lots of people, weight training wasn't the answer for me. The doctor told me that I had to go down to the gym and start lifting free weights and I thought, No, thank you. I'm not going to do that. I worried about dropping them and injuring myself. They're hard on the back; they're not portable so you can't take them anywhere; you're just kind of held hostage by the gym or the weight bench. I'm a real advocate of resistance training using heavy elastic bands. It's a whole lot safer; it gives you the same kind of results, and it's portable. I'm sure you've seen the rubber band products where you hold the handles and stretch the band until your muscles have to resist. So I developed a product called the Gym Bag based on that principle. My band is a maximum forty pounds of resistance. In other words, it's the same as lifting forty pounds of free weights; it's just using a resistance band. The way it works is that when you're pulling and stretching the band, the more you pull it, the more weight is on it. In other words, if you pull the band out to its maximum, it would be equivalent to lifting forty pounds of free weight on a barbell.

An analogy is that if we have a rubber band and we stretch it and then we let it go back in, there's resistance on the band. But when you make it a forty-pound resistant band, then, of course, you have to pull a whole lot harder, which works the muscle groups in the specific area you are trying to affect.

I wanted to develop something from which I could get the benefit of resistance or strength training and not be restricted to my house or the gym or wherever. So I put the forty-pound band with cushioned handles into a little

6-inch bag, and now I can do all the things I need to do, whether I'm home or on the road, to keep my bones strong and to keep myself in as good shape as possible inside and out. I use the band (and the workout only takes eight minutes) in conjunction with my BodyFlex exercises.

The important thing is to find a weight-bearing exercise—lifting weights or resistance training—that suits you and that you will do regularly. Buying the equipment and keeping it on a shelf doesn't count. Do something to keep your bones safe for the second half of your life.

Do you need any other workouts beyond BodyFlex? I feel that BodyFlex is a full program on its own for anyone below age forty. But as we start into our forties, it's time to add a strength or resistance program. However, if you're looking to be a body builder or have a body builder's body, then BodyFlex is not the program for you. What we end up with when we do BodyFlex solely is more of a dancer's body—no excess body fat, lean and limber, defined and flexible. In my opinion, a ballet dancer is the most physically fit person there is. And all the workouts really consist of is movement, bending, stretching, and breathing exercises. Many of the ballet dancers do the Pilates system of deep breathing (named for the person who created it). I taught some dancers in the Houston Ballet the BodyFlex program and they told me that it just kicked the butt out of Pilates. BodyFlex is so much more advanced in elongating muscle, which tones us and gives us range of motion.

So feed your body well and keep your bones strong, and you'll find that the benefits of BodyFlex are like the Energizer bunny—they keep going and going and going and going . . .

9

The Picture of Health

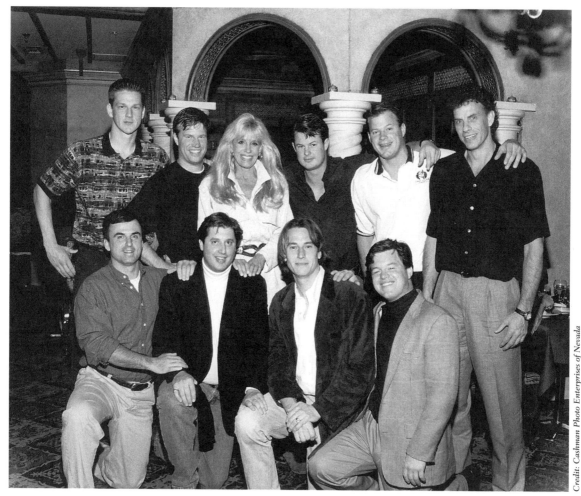

BodyFlex isn't just for women. Rich men, poor men,
beggarmen, thieves, doctors, lawyers . . .

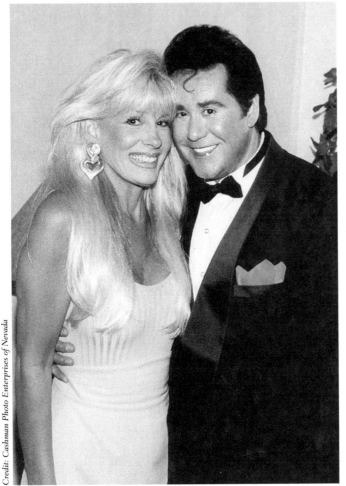

Over the last fifteen years I have received thousands of letters from people BodyFlex has helped. I would like to share a few of these testimonials with you, as well as some pictures of me with a few of my clients, from the famous to the average American. Now you know why I take pride in saying that all my friends are losers.

Dear Ms. Childers,

My heartfelt thanks for saving my sanity! BodyFlex eliminated my stress and 11½ inches in just two weeks!

I was introduced to the program at the worst time in my life. During that time, I was caring for my mother who was dying of breast cancer, raising

. . . Indian chief. The top tomahawk in show business and one talented and terrific guy, Wayne Newton is also a BodyFlex fan.

my daughter, and working a high-stress job that required 65–70 hours a week. While trying so hard to balance everything, I started feeling like my life was crumbling around me. It was during that time that BodyFlex came into my life. I still can't believe what it's done for me, and only in 15 minutes a day! All my cares, stress, and anxiety started to go away, and I started feeling like I could manage my life again. I have more energy and look physically fit.

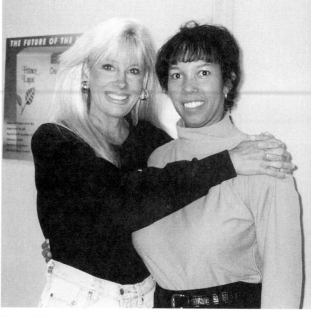

BodyFlex once a day helps keep the doctor away. Thank goodness lovely nurse R. June Young has gotten with the program and taken intensive care of herself.

BodyFlex is now a way of life for me, and I wish everyone could experience how wonderful it makes you feel. Thank you, Greer, for sharing your program and making me a happy person.

Sincerely,
R. June Young

Dear Greer,
I wanted to take a moment to share with you how much your program, BodyFlex, has affected my life.

Due to your time and generosity, I have been able to conquer an area of my life that has caused years of personal frustration. I never had the kind of confidence in my ability to maintain my figure the way I wanted to see myself until now. I used to get up every day and stress over how much and what I should be eating, and then beat myself to death in the gym, only to find my size was going up instead of down.

Since I started doing BodyFlex I have slimmed down and people refer to me as being thin and trim. Not only do I feel much better, but I look better and I am free from the diet/exercise yo-yo syndrome.

Greer, you will be immortal in my life, and I thank God every day that I had the privilege of meeting you and BodyFlex.

Love,
Carolyn Vanzlow

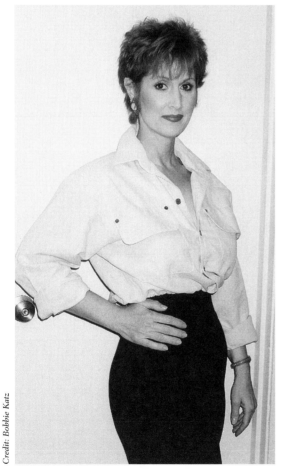

Credit: Bobbie Katz

Dear Greer,

When I was a child, I had an abundance of energy; after puberty, my metabolism slowed down dramatically and I no longer had the energy necessary for daily living . . . in my thirties and forties I would sleep up to twelve hours a day and still feel like I had not slept at all. I was beginning to despair and had depression all the time, causing me to sleep even more. I had no joy in doing the things I love. No energy for anything extra; weekends were spent resting just to be able to work during the week. Now after one month of

Mirror, mirror on the wall, who's one of the slimmest of them all? Skin-care consultant Carolyn Vanzlow, a BodyFlex success, knows that beauty is more than skin deep.

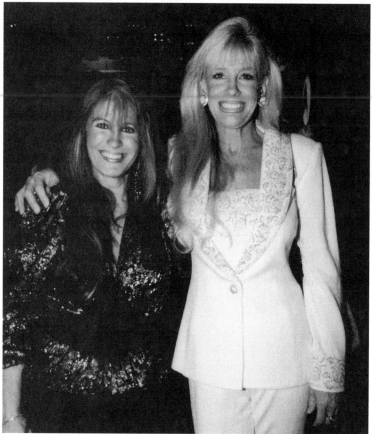

Credit: Tony Scodwell

No ands, ifs, or butts about it, Greer and Bobbie are friends to their ends, which are considerably smaller and firmer than they used to be.

doing BodyFlex faithfully every day, I have an abundance of energy again. I feel like I'm ten years old; I only need to sleep six to seven hours a night *and I sleep deep and restful*, waking up with the energy to do my BodyFlex and go, go, go, go, go, go into the day. Thank you for developing BodyFlex and giving me my life back.

    Linda M. Ohman Clark

Dear Greer,

. . . I *hate*, absolutely *hate*, getting hot and sweaty, so I have always hated exercise, except for swimming and now, except for BodyFlex. I don't have to change clothes, although sometimes I will take off my pumps. I have four pieces of equipment that I have collected over a period of 2 years that I have been using with precious little to show for 20 minutes a day—increase in endurance and strength but weight and inches *the same*. Fed up? You bet! In fact, I stopped exercising back in September.

Then I saw BodyFlex and ordered it, figuring what the_ _ _ _. When it came, I saved the box figuring I would send it back when it didn't work. After all, it *looked* too easy! It *sounded* too easy! No huffing and puffing and getting all sweaty! What sort of exercise was this? I burned the box last week. I'm not sending this back! Here's why:

	Starting	1st week	2nd week	3rd week
Upper abs	36	35	35	34
Waist	36	36	35	33½
Lower abs	45	42	42	40
Hips	47	47	45	43
Thighs	28	27	25	24

Now, in my third week of BodyFlex, I have lost 17½ inches! By the way, I am 5-foot-2 and weigh 163 pounds. I'm fifty years old with two girls—19 and 13. I'm a substitute teacher in all subject areas, although social studies and science are my favorite subjects. I'm going to my thirtieth junior college class reunion at the end of April. It will be interesting to see what the inches will be down to by then.

Looking forward to seeing more of you on HSN.

Sincerely,

Joan Sugg

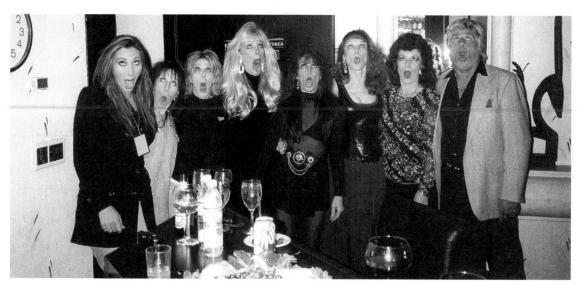

My buddies and I doing the Lion. Here us roar!

Dear Greer,

I want to say a BIG thank you for those wonderful tapes. In 1984, I had total knee replacement in both of my knees. In 1993, I broke my right ankle and damaged the prosthesis in my right knee and had to have it replaced. Since 1984, I had not been able to kneel on my knees. Since using your tapes, I am now able to get on my knees. I started by using a pillow to kneel on—now I don't even need the pillow. These exercises have given me so much mobility and energy. As far as the inches lost, I have lost, but my main concern is what the program has done for my mobility. All the therapy I have had didn't do as much good as these tapes. Thank you, thank you, thank you!

   Helen T.

Dear Greer,

I just have to write and tell you how much I enjoy the BodyFlex system.

I'm 33, married, and have two boys, ages 12 and 8.

I have enclosed a copy of my loss *so far*. I was amazed at my first week loss of 15¼ inches. But in four weeks, I have lost 38½ inches and have gone from a tight 18 to a loose 16!

I have never had more energy. I get up at 5:30–6:00 A.M. every morning (I used to drop out of bed at 7:15 A.M.).

I just wanted to tell you thank you for changing my life. God bless you.

Sincerely,
Melanie Kelly

Dear Ms. Childers,

I just wanted to write to you to let you know that you have changed my life!

After a lifetime of being fat and trying anything I could do to lose weight, I've finally found something that seems to be working—your tapes!

I purchased them at the end of January and, to date [April], I have lost twenty-seven pounds! I have really been watching what I eat along with your video and I had to tell you that yours is the first exercise technique I can live with. I have all kinds of exercise equipment in my basement that I got sick of using, but BodyFlex is so quick and simple that I look forward to doing it. You are a godsend.

At first, I didn't lose a lot of inches, but I figured I was so far overweight that I would just have to work a little harder at it. Little by little, I'm losing it and it feels great! I still have a long way to go, but with BodyFlex, I am confident that I will reach my goal.

. . . Anyway, thank you again for the best exercise video

I've ever seen. I'm telling all my friends to buy it. We're all in our mid-forties and it's hard to find a system we can live with. You have helped many people and may God bless you and your family. With BodyFlex, I think my dream of someday being a normal size will come true.

With much appreciation and love,
Linda Brydges

Dear Greer,
I wanted to write and share my excitement for BodyFlex. Yes, it is like no other.

When I first played the instructional tape, I was shocked to see the deep breathing. But now I find myself deep breathing at work when I'm alone in the elevator and while driving to and from work. It gives me more energy thru the day.

Even my sixteen-year-old daughter Carissa is using the BodyFlex tapes.

. . . I do thank you for sharing your system with me. . . .

Respectfully,
Christine J. Wilson

Dear Greer,
I have been going to sit down and write you for some time (even to the extent of writing notes in my head to you), but never get down to doing it, so here I am. Finally! First of all, thank you, thank you, thank you for making up the two videos, which you presented on Home Shopping. I do them faithfully each and every day, like a ritual, and have noted GREAT RESULTS (so have my family and friends). I'm only sorry that I didn't take my measurements BEFORE starting, but it is evidenced in my clothes and the way in which they fit NOW!

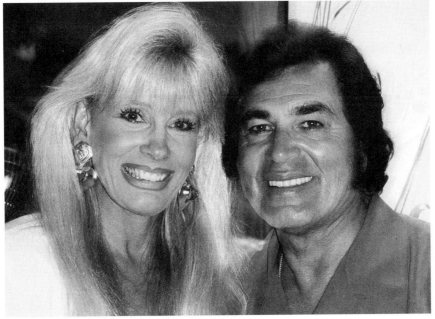

Credit: Bobbie Katz

Engelbert Humperdinck is my most gorgeous client, an international superstar, and a great guy besides.

I am a woman sixty-seven years old, who unfortunately has had a lot of surgery, which involved the opening and closing of my abdomen. Therefore, that coupled with my having had two pregnancies have made my stomach without the elasticity most people have; however, you are MY HERO, STRENGTH, AND A REAL VISIBLE; I AM TRULY INSPIRED BY YOU AND YOUR STORY. . . .

. . . Last Tuesday, I got the ULTIMATE compliment, Greer, when the gym teacher in our senior center asked me to demonstrate what I have been doing to the class!

. . . You have motivated me BEYOND my wildest dreams. You are my INSPIRATION!

Thank you and God bless you,

Margie Gray

Dear Ms. Childers,

I suffer from Epstein-Barr virus, which causes chronic fatigue. Normal exercise only intensifies the fatigue, and stress always causes the virus to act up. I was told that your program had helped others and could help me. I have to admit that I was skeptical but decided that I had nothing to lose by giving it a try for one month.

Praise God, your program has increased my energy level beyond belief, allowing me to work for the last six months without having to go home, fall into bed to sleep for twelve hours, only to wake up seemingly more tired

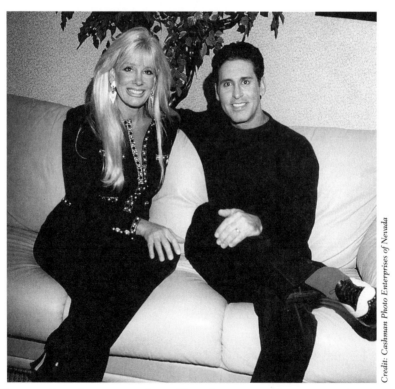

Credit: Cashman Photo Enterprises of Nevada

Danny Gans is a man of a million faces—and one great body. He was named Entertainer of the Year in Las Vegas and is the only client I've ever had with a waist smaller than mine.

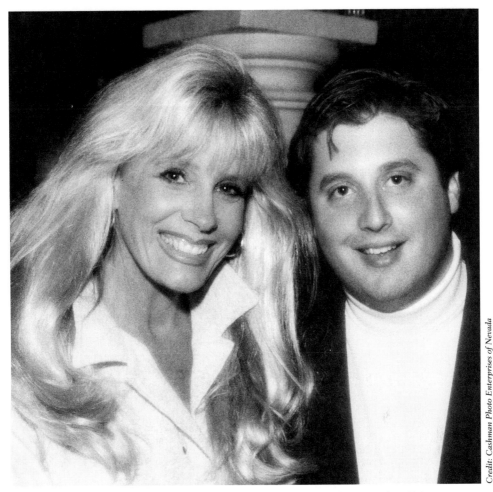

Credit: Cashman Photo Enterprises of Nevada

Skip Borghese is a real Prince of a guy . . . grandson to the Princess
Marcella Borghese of Italy and a BodyFlex client, too.

than when I fell into bed. Also, for the past three months,
I have been under much stress caused by a separation
and still I have been able to work and care for my home.

I have lived with Epstein-Barr virus for over ten years
and know how my body is affected and how it reacted to
exercise and stress in the past. I now have more energy
than I have had in over ten years and I *know* that it is be-

cause of your BodyFlex program. I have and will continue to recommend it to everybody I know.

Thank you again for all that your tapes have done for me.

Sincerely,

Rhonda Allen

P.S. I have also lost 8½ inches. What a deal!

10

Be a Loser

*D*id you ever think you could feel terrific about being called a loser?

Well, I want you to be able to have the feeling of pride that comes with being called a *big* loser, one who is getting rid of those areas of ugly, unwanted fat and flab literally in one blow and having her dress sizes drop like flies.

*G*et Motivated, Stay Motivated

Here's what you have to do to be a loser: You have to make losing and getting in shape a priority. Sound easy? Well, here's some reinforcing steps. Get up in the morning, go into the bathroom, take your nightgown off, and look at yourself in the mirror. Look at yourself full face then take another mirror and turn around and get the back view— take a good look at your butt, your legs, your back flab. This will either make you feel a little sick (luckily, you're already in the bathroom) or give you a big clue that you need to motivate yourself each morning to do something about it . . . besides inflicting more harm on yourself (it was Miss Scarlet, in the buff, in the bathroom, with a shower tie). I know all about it. Looking at myself on a daily basis was the only motivation that ever worked for me.

Now start doing BodyFlex and look at yourself, in the buff, in the bathroom, front and back, every morning. After about four or five days, you're going to start to say, "You know what? I don't look so bad. My thighs don't look so bumpy. My stomach doesn't look so poochy. My butt doesn't look so lumpy." You're going to see visible results day by day, with your own eyes, as you look at your reflection. And you'll see them in the first seven days. What more of a daily remotivator do you need to spur you on to do fifteen minutes of BodyFlex?

No More Excuses

Take a close look at every excuse you've ever given yourself on why you don't have fifteen minutes a day to spend giving yourself the gift of health and vitality. Tell yourself no more excuses.

I want you to be a loser as much as you want to be a loser. And I'm going to help you get results in spite of yourself. You can try and prove me wrong. You can go into this with an attitude of "Well, I'll show her it won't work. Let me just do it each day." Frankly, my dears, I don't give a darn what your philosophy is. Because for once in your life, it doesn't matter if you believe it or like it or hate it or hate me or love me. The program works in spite of it all because it's a matter of physics.

As I've said repeatedly, we all have to start somewhere. We're not looking to be elite gymnasts. We're not looking to be world-class athletes. We just want more energy. We want to look good. We want to be fit. We want to tighten up our bodies and we don't want to carry an extra twenty, thirty, forty, fifty pounds of fat around with us. If you've never exercised, especially if you're older, maybe you can't do fifteen minutes the first day. You know what you do? You do what you can. If you can only do five minutes the first day, that's okay. Because the next day you'll be able to do six minutes. And two days later, you'll be able to do ten minutes. And down the line, you'll be able to do fourteen minutes. Pretty soon you'll be able to do fifteen minutes. Everybody has his or her own level that they have to start at. Just don't be afraid to start. Because if you don't do it at all, then you really have something to be afraid of!

A lot of people out there have some kind of limitation—they're in a wheelchair, bedridden, or on crutches; they've got arthritis, fibromyalgia, Epstein-Barr, on and on and on. If this is your problem, it's the same philosophy: You can do what you can, that's all you can do. There are people who want us to hit the ground running—I look at TV and bust up laughing. Those walkers and treadmills and ab rollers and other exercise gizmos that do everything but make coffee are a joke. A lot of my clients can't even put one foot in front of the other because their knees hurt so bad or they have ankle problems or their backs hurt.

As I've said, the beauty of this program is that you can adapt it to whatever level you're at, whether you are a high-performance athlete or a convalescent. If you are bedridden and you want to be fit and look better, there's been practically nothing for you up until now. But what you're going to do is take baby steps to fitness . . . Get your doctor's okay, then just do a little bit each and every day. A little bit is better than nothing. And if you can do a little bit today, next week you can do a little more, the next week a little bit more, the next week more, so you can progress and get better and better. I repeat, you have to start somewhere. If you don't, you're going nowhere.

Many people who suffer from all sorts of limitations will call me and say, "I can't do this because my back hurts, I can't do this because my knees hurt," etc. And I tell them, be creative. Do this program on your bed. If you can't even do it on your bed, then just do the breathing. The breathing alone will give you a tremendous amount of benefit, from energy to a stronger immune system. When you are feeling stronger, maybe you can take the next step and just do one position. And then after a couple of weeks, do another one.

Total Wellness and a Great Waistline

One question all of you out there need to ask yourselves is, if you keep going the way you are going, making no changes, do you think that in thirty days from now, you're going to look and feel better or look and feel worse? I think you already know the answer to that. You definitely won't be any better, but it's very possible that you'll be worse because if you make no changes, you'll get no results.

If you don't want to do BodyFlex, that's okay. But if you don't do this, what *are* you going to do? I believe that we have to take as many preventative steps as possible where our health is concerned, to help ourselves. The field of alternative medicine is growing by leaps and bounds. Insurance companies are now covering alternative remedies. And 40 percent of the general public is now looking to it as an alternative to Western medicine. No longer can Western medicine turn a blind eye to this holistic way of taking care of our bodies. There's too much research and too much proof that it works to dispute it any longer.

Alternative medicine, of which I consider BodyFlex a part, focuses on a holistic approach and preventative care. Western medical doctors are trained to treat specific diseases. They are not trained to promote preventative care. And they are not looking at the big picture of overall health.

I talk a lot about slim waists and firm thighs, but my real commitment to the folks who do BodyFlex is to help them achieve total wellness. I want to help you take every preventative step you can instead of waiting until you get some life-threatening disease and then sitting back and wondering if there was something you could have done to help get your immune system functioning at its optimum level. Why wait? The time to take action is before something happens. The time to put a smoke alarm in the house is before the house burns to the ground.

In this book, you have read about the benefits oxygenation gives the body. We know oxygen does two very important things: It burns body fat, and it produces energy. Wouldn't it be great if we could go to the store and order three bottles of energy and two bottles of fat-burning elixir? BodyFlex provides both.

For many years, you have wanted a new figure. You have wanted new vitality, an improved feeling of health. Conversely, over the years, perhaps you have learned to rationalize, to accept less. Maybe you have developed an unrealistic self-image based on indulgence in unsatisfactory living.

To break these unwanted habits and let the real you emerge, I suggest that you spend some time with yourself imagining how you really want to live and be, picturing and feeling what it would be like to attain the goals you want. Imagine yourself being healthy and confident and vigorous. Then imagine yourself doing things differently. Imagine yourself playing tennis. Imagine yourself dancing. Imagine yourself in a more powerful position. Imagine yourself succeeding in all these new images. Nurture yourself. Give yourself the kind of care, support, and encouragement that you give to your loved ones.

I have found that the most successful people in the BodyFlex program are those who have been able to adjust to the new images that flow from this program. The fact of the matter is, the people who desire most, believe most, and consciously put forth the effort to strive for these new images are the ones who end up changing their lives the most. So, take BodyFlex to its full potential. Change your physiology and thus your psychology. Change your beliefs about yourself and your belief in your limitations.

To reiterate what Burton Goldberg, best-selling author of *Alternative Medicine: The Definitive Guide,* says in his interview with me and my cowriter: "BodyFlex is a total package for total health and is one of the most incredibly inexpensive things you can do for yourself to control your own destiny. Using the knowledge on these pages, you can get well and stay well."

Oxygen is truly the non-medical miracle. And BodyFlex is the way to get the benefits of this miracle.

$\mathcal{T}$ he Loser of a Lifetime

So don't say no to exercise. Win the losing battle against low energy and lack of fitness. Be the loser of a lifetime with BodyFlex. Your lifetime.

Bobbie Katz has a B.S. in communications and theater from Temple University in Philadelphia and has been a professional journalist for the last twenty-eight years. Since 1986, she has been a celebrity interviewer and feature writer for several national publications, and among her recent credits is a cover story on Roseanne for *First* magazine and two features on Las Vegas entertainment for a special edition of *Variety*. She has also served as the entertainment editor for several national magazines based in Atlantic City and Las Vegas, and for the last three years has been a Vegas-based correspondent covering the Las Vegas entertainment scene for the Sunday Calendar section of the *Los Angeles Times*. She has interviewed hundreds of big-name celebrities of stage, screen, and TV for print, radio (she had her own radio show), and videotape, many of them numerous times.

Ms. Katz has also been doing the BodyFlex program for the last two and a half years, having gone from a size 12–14 to a size 1–3, where she remains today, in ninety days using this exercise technique. She has written magazine articles about Ms. Childers and is a leading advocate of the BodyFlex program, giving first-hand testimony as to how well the program works and how it has changed her life.